SOPHIA LOPEZ

LEAN AND GREEN COOKBOOK

100% for vegetarian

MANAGE YOUR FIGURE
EASY, TASTY, AND HEALTHY RECIPES
TO LOSE WEIGHT

BONUS NEW VEGAN RECIPES

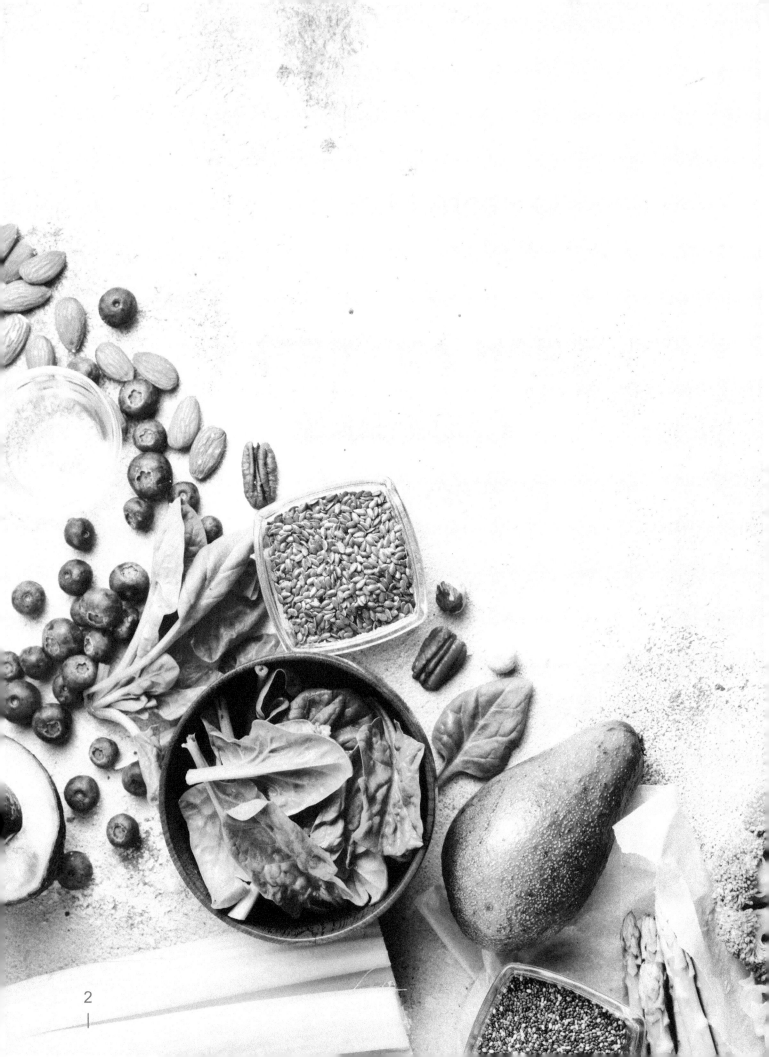

TABLE OF CONTENTS

TABLE OF CONTENTS

various sources. Please consult a licensed professional before attempting any techniques outlined in this book.

By reading this document, the reader agrees that under no circumstances is the author responsible for any losses, direct or indirect, which are incurred as a result of the use of information contained within this document, including, but not limited to, — errors, omissions, or inaccuracies.

INTRODUCTION

Have you heard of the Lean and Green Diet, and now you wish to know more about it? Are you vegetarian or vegan and you are looking for recipes to lose weight? Here you are! In this cookbook, you'll find several easy, tasty, and healthy recipes to manage your figure.

The Lean and Green diet is for individuals who wish to lose weight because of its low-calorie approach. It's suitable for individuals living a busy lifestyle. Inside this book you will find everything you ever wanted to learn about it, how it works, about lean and green foods, and last but not least with just vegetarian and vegan recipes.

This cookbook is focused on the idea of making quick meals that are as healthy as delicious. Most of us come home late and we're so exhausted that we sacrifice our meals to focus on seemingly more important things. I share recipes that will take you from ten minutes to less the one hour to make it but with any compromises on flavor.

More and more people are pursuing vegetarianism and veganism, we all know that eating more vegetarian and vegan foods is good not only for our health but also for the environment and our wallets.

After you read this book, you will make wise decisions that will substantially benefit your health. Everything you need to know about the Lean and Green Diet, plus lots of healthy recipes, environmentally and, animals responsible.

I wish you a healthy life and enjoy your meal!

Sophia Lopez

WHAT IS THE LEAN AND GREEN DIET?

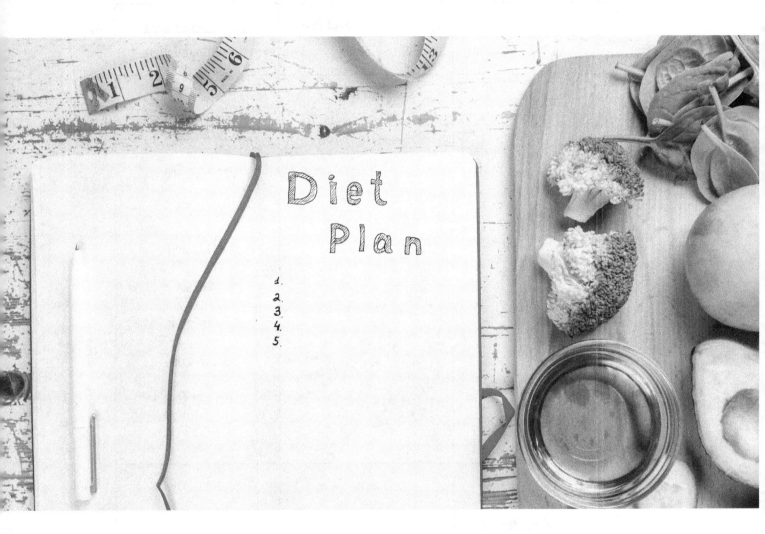

The Lean and Green Diet encourages people to limit the number of calories that they should take daily. Under this program, dieters are encouraged to consume between 800 and 1000 calories daily.

For this to be possible, dieters are encouraged to opt for healthier food items and meal replacements. There are currently three variations of the Lean and Green plan that one can choose according to one's needs.

How Nutritious Is Lean and Green Diet

	Optimal Weight 5&1 Plan	Federal Government Recommendation
Calories	800-1,000	Men 19-25: 2,800 26-45: 2,600 46-65: 2,400 65+: 2,200 Women 19-25: 2,200 26-50: 2,000 51+: 1,800
Total fat % of Calorie Intake	20%	20%-35%
Total Carbohydrates % of Calorie Intake	40%	45%-65%
Sugars	10%-20%	N/A

Fiber	25 g – 30 g	Men
		19-30: 34 g.
		31-50: 31 g.
		51+: 28 g.
		Women
		19-30: 28 g.
		31-50: 25 g.
		51+: 22 g.
Protein	40%	10%-35%
Sodium	Under 2,300 mg	Under 2,300 mg.
Potassium	Average 3,000 mg	At least 4,700 mg.
Calcium	1,000 mg – 1,200 mg	Men
		1,000 mg.
		Women
		19-50: 1,000 mg.
		51+: 1,200 mg.

How to Start This Diet

The Lean and Green Diet comprises different phases. For the sake of those who are new to this diet, below are some of the things that you need to know, especially when you are still starting with this diet regimen.

Initial Steps

During this phase, people are encouraged to consume 800 to 1,000 calories to help you shed off at least 12 pounds within the next 12 weeks. For instance, if you are following the 5&1 Plan, you need to eat 1 meal every 2 or 3 hours and include a 30-minute moderate workout on most days of your week. You need to consume not more than 100 grams of Carbohydrates daily during this phase.

Further, consuming the Lean and Green meals is highly encouraged. It involves eating 5 to 7 ounces of cooked lean proteins, three servings of non-starchy vegetables, and two healthy fats. This phase also encourages the dieter to include one optional snack per day, such as 1/2 cup sugar-free gelatin, three celery sticks, and 12 ounces nuts. Aside from these things, below are other things that you need to remember when following this phase:

- Make sure that the portion size recommendations are for cooked weight and not the raw -weight of your ingredients
- Opt for meals that are baked, grilled, broiled, or poached. Avoid frying foods, as this will increase your calorie intake.
- Eat at least two servings of fish rich in Omega-3 fatty acids. These include fishes like tuna, salmon, trout, mackerel, herring, and other cold-water fishes.
- Follow the program even when you are dining out. Keep in mind that drinking alcohol is discouraged when following this plan.

Maintenance Phase

As soon as you have achieved your desired weight, the next phase is the transition stage. It is a 6-week stage that involves increasing your calorie intake to 1,550 per day. This is also the phase when you can add more varieties into your meal, such as whole grains, low-fat dairy, and fruits.

After six weeks, you can now move into the 3&3 Lean and Green Diet plan, so you are required to eat three Lean and Green meals and 3 Fueling foods.

Lean & Green Meals When You're Dining Out

You have straightforward instructions for what, where, and how much to consume when you're on the Lean and Green 5 & 1 Program. So, what about going out while you are on your plan? With balanced Lean & Green Meals, or healthy choices for the Transition and Maintenance periods, you will remain on track almost everywhere you go. Just a bit of preparation and innovation is what it requires. Many restaurants have options that, with a bit of change, are consistent with the system or can be. The vital thing to remember is that asking your waiter questions regarding the "customization" of your meal is all correct. Most places will be more than willing to satisfy specific needs and can provide free, or with a minor extra fee, alternative replacements.

Check the guidelines for the appropriate beverages. Simple water is still suitable; use a lime slice and ice or your chosen Flavor Infuser to spruce it up. Stick to drinks that are calorie-free, such as diet drinks, sugar-free tea, coffee, fizzy water, or seltzer that is salt-free.

Diet would not encourage the consumption of alcohol in people who are in the program's weight loss phase, particularly if you have diabetes. Alcohol not only contributes empty calories but facilitates exhaustion and may reduce willpower, reducing one's approach to the desire to order bad foods. In comparison, the impact of alcohol on those adopting a reduced-calorie food program will be felt more easily and can raise the risk of associated side effects with alcohol use.

Tips to Stay on Track Before Your Dine Out

1. Be Ready, Be Willing

Good eating will become a common routine once you understand what a balanced diet feels like. You would just be aware of exactly what to do when a sudden dining chance introduces itself.

2. Ask Yourself These Questions:

- What will I do if anyone causes me a tough time making my decisions?
- What will I do if I haven't been to this place before?
- What will I do if they do have my beloved dessert/dish?

You would be well able to cope with them with ease by simply "talking yourself through" the scenarios you are likely to experience at the restaurant. Eating out is fun and hassle-free with just a little planning.

3. Research Menus

Many diners have online menus, and some also print their dishes with nutritional values. If there is no information there and the restaurant is close, try pulling up for an early look. Using the Lean & Green dietary criteria as a reference, make better decisions when nutrition knowledge is available. Taking a look at the deals in advance helps you to take your time and allows safe, conscientious decisions. Without feeling pressured or self-conscious, you'll recognize what to order once you're comfortable. If you can't seem to find one that is perfect for your program phase, inquire! Most restaurants under the Lean & Green meal standards are able to satisfy basic demands for something.

You should feel secure in inquiring about healthier foods, much like you will not think twice before buying anything unique for those with food intolerances or other nutritional requirements. Know the goal is to feel better regarding your nutritious decisions.

4. Choose Supportive Companions

Often, it's just as important to acknowledge who you hang with as where you hang. Make sure your friends are respectful of you and your activities the first few occasions you consume in a diner after beginning the diet path. Soon, no matter the business, you'll be relaxed enough to make the correct choices.

THE LEAN & GREEN FOODS

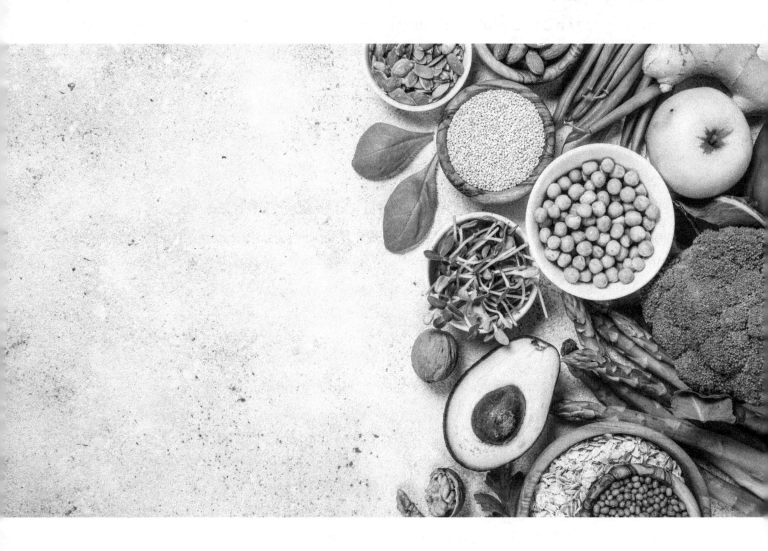

Depending on the options for lean protein, a Lean & Green meal contains 5 to 7 oz. of some healthy lean protein that is thoroughly cooked along with three serves of veggies that are specifically non-starchy and low-crab in nature and two parts of the good fats. Any time of day, eat your Lean & Green food, however, fits better with your schedule.

Use the below Lean & Green Meal Nutrient Criteria to better lead your decisions, whether you are eating out or measuring your intake:

Healthy Fats

Integrate up to two portions of good fats with your Lean & Green meal every day. Good fats are essential because they help to digest vitamins such as A, D, E, and K from your body. They even support the proper functioning of the gallbladder. There should be 5 grams of overall fat and fewer than 5 g of carbohydrates in a serving of good fat. Below, you will find a bunch of healthy fat options.

The "Lean" Part of Your Lean & Green Meal

Below are a few of the helpful tips for choosing your "Lean" protein. These portion size guidelines are for cooked weight only, not raw.

- Choose grilled, roasted, steamed, or poached meat, not fried.
- Prefer to eat at least two portions of fish (salmon, cod, sardines, trout, or herring) high in omega-3 fatty acids a week.
- Feel free to use choices like tofu and kimchi that are meat-free.

Choose from the collection that will be listed below the required single serving of any meat. We've sorted protein into the leanest, leaner, and lean choices. For the Ideal Weight 5 & 1 Program, all methods are suitable; this merely lets you make better food decisions. You will use the following nutritional details for any protein alternative, not on the list, to decide whether it is suitable for the Lean and Green system.

Lean & Green Meal Nutritional Criteria

- Calories = 250-400 Kcal
- 20 grams of carbohydrates (preferably < 15 g)
- Greater than or equal to 25 grams of Protein
- 10-20 grams of fat

"Lean" Part of the Lean & Green Meal

- 180-300 Calories
- Carbohydrates <= 15 g
- Protein >= 25 g
- For fat, refer to the groups of specific proteins below

Leanest Protein Options

- Pick 5 oz. Cooked part of 10 g - 20 g of total fat with no extra Good Fat portion.
- Fish: trout, salmon (Bluefin steak), halibut, mackerel, farmed catfish
- Lean beef: roast, barbecue, minced
- Mutton
- Pork chop or tenderloin pork
- Turkey meatballs or other protein which is approximately 85%-94% lean meat
- Dark meat: poultry or turkey

Your choices for meat-free protein are:

- 15 oz. extra firm or medium tofu
- 3 complete eggs (up to 2 days a week)
- Four ounces of lowered-fat or skim cheese (3-6 g fat per oz.) or 1 cup shredded.
- 8 oz. • (1 cup) Ricotta part-skim cheese (2-3 g of fat per oz.)
- Five ounces. of tempeh

Leanest Protein Options

- Pick 7 oz. Cooked section with 0-4 g net fat and 2 Good fat portions incorporated.
- Fish: flounder, shrimp, salmon, grouper, orange roughy, haddock, tuna, wild catfish (fresh meat or canned in brine)
- Shellfish: lobster, shrimp, scallops, crabs
- Game meat: moose, cows, deer
- Ground turkey or other protein: roughly 98 percent lean meat

Your choices for meat-free protein are:

- 14 whites of egg
- 2 cups of fresh egg whites or fresh egg replacer
- Five oz. of seitan
- 1 and a half cups (12 ounces) 1% cottage cheese
- 12 ounces of nonfat regular Greek yogurt (about 15 g carb per 12 ounces) (0 percent)

Leaner Protein Options

- Pick 6 oz. Cooked part with 5 to 9 g of fat content and one good fat serving attached. Turkey meatballs or any other protein: 95%-97% lean meat
- Turkey: Light meat
- Poultry: breast or white meat, stripped of skin
- Fish: salmon, shrimp, halibut

Your choices for meat-free protein are:

- 2 entire eggs and one cup of liquid egg replacement
- 1 1/2 cups (12 ounces) 2% cottage cheese
- 12 ounces of any good low-fat (2%) regular Greek yogurt (which is approximately 15 g carb per 12 oz.)
- 2 full eggs and four whites of eggs

Healthy Fat Servings

Around 5g of fat and much less than 5g of carbs can be included in a good fat portion. Attach 0 2 regular Good Fat Portions depending on the Lean Options:

- 1 teaspoon of oil (any sort)
- 1 tablespoon of normal, low-carb dressing for the salad
- 2 teaspoons lessened-fat, low-carb dressing for a salad
- 5-10 green or black olives
- 1 1/2 oz. Avocado
- 1/3 oz. Simple food items, such as peanuts, pistachios, or almonds
- 1 tablespoon of regular seeds, like chia seeds, flaxseed, pumpkin seeds, or sesame seeds
- Standard butter, ghee, or mayo for 1/2 tablespoons

The "Green" Part of Your Lean & Green Meal

For each one of the Lean & Green meals, pick three meals from the Green list of options below. We also grouped the choices for vegetables into higher, moderate, and lower amounts of carbohydrates. On the Optimum Weight 5 & 1 Schedule, each is acceptable; the guide lets you make better decisions regarding food.

From the Green Choices List, select three servings:

- One portion = 1/2 cup of vegetables with less than or equal to 25 calories and less than or just about 5 g of carbohydrate (until otherwise indicated).

(NOTE: All vegetables encourage healthier eating. However, we omit the highest possible carb veggies (such as broccoli, maize, peas, potatoes, onions, asparagus, and green beans) in the Optimum Weight 5 & 1 Strategy to boost the outcomes. We urge you to use more veggies for long-term wellbeing after you've reached your healthier weight).

Lower Carbohydrate Greens

- One cup: collard (fresh/raw), endive, cabbage, mustard greens, lettuce (fresh/raw), spring mix, watercress, scallions (raw), green leaf, zucchini squash, broccoli, romaine.
- Half a cup of Arugula, cucumbers, celery, radishes, jalapeño (raw), sprouts (mung bean, alfalfa), white mushrooms, escarole, Swiss chard (raw), turnip greens, nopales, bok choy (cooked).

Moderate Carbohydrate Greens

- Half a cup: asparagus, eggplant, summer squash (zucchini or scallop), broccoli, lettuce, roasted spinach, fennel seed, portobello mushrooms, cauliflower, etc.
- Higher Carbohydrate Greens
- Half a cup: Turnips, cooked Swiss chard, cooked chayote squash, cooked mustard or collard leaves, red cabbage, broccoli, jicama, cooked squash, cooked green or wax beans, cooked kohlrabi, cooked leeks, cooked peppers, raw scallions, palm hearts, cooked summer squash (crookneck), cooked tomatoes, okra, cooked spaghetti squash.

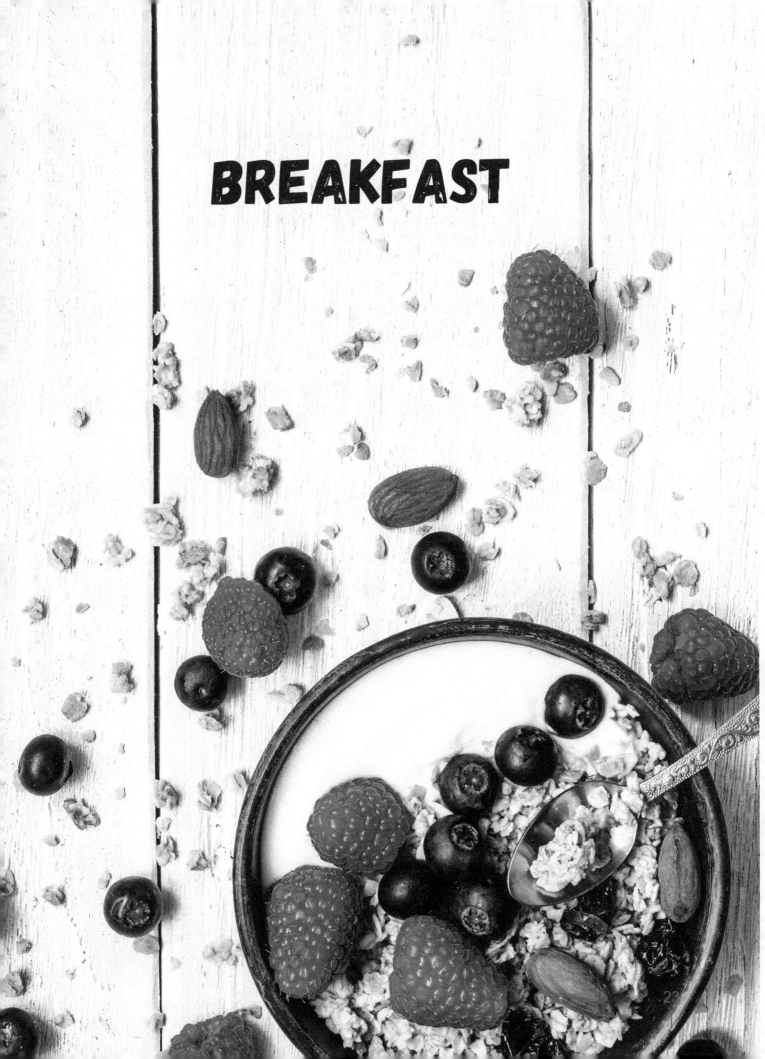

BREAKFAST

GREEK YOGURT BREAKFAST BARK

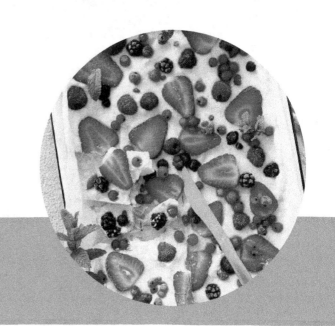

PREP. TIME: 5' · COOK TIME: 5' · SERVINGS: 2

INGREDIENTS

- 12 ounces plain low-fat Greek yogurt
- 2 packets zero-calorie sugar substitute
- 1 mix red berry

DIRECTIONS

01 Line an 8x8 baking dish with non-stick foil. Set aside.

02 In a bowl, combine the Greek yogurt and sugar substitute.
Spread the Greek yogurt mixture into the prepared baking dish and sprinkle with mix red berry

03 Put in the freezer for 5 hours until the bark is hard.
Break the bark with a sharp knife into smaller pieces.

NUTRITIONAL FACTS

- Calories: 198 Cal,
- Protein: 11.1 g,
- Carbohydrates: 31.2 g,
- Fat: 3.1 g,
- Sugar: 15.4 g

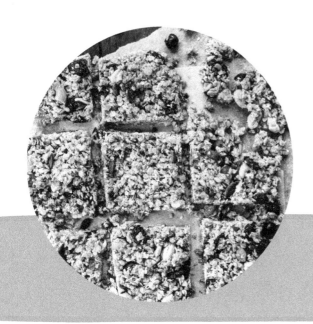

QUICKIE HONEY NUT GRANOLA

PREP. TIME: 10' · COOK TIME: 20' · SERVINGS: 6

DIRECTIONS

01 Preheat the oven to 325°F. Line a large, rimmed baking sheet with parchment paper. In a large skillet, combine the oats, almonds, salt, and cinnamon. Turn the heat to medium-high and cook, often stirring till toast, about 6 minutes.

02 While the oat mixture is toasting, in a microwave-safe bowl, combine the apricots, flaxseed, honey, and oil. Microwave on high for about 1 minute, or until very hot and just beginning to bubble.

03 Stir the vanilla into the honey mixture, then pour it over the oat mixture in the skillet. Stir well.

04 Spread out the granola on the prepared baking sheet. Bake for 15 minutes, until lightly browned. Remove from the oven and cool completely. Break the granola into small pieces, and store in an airtight container in the refrigerator for up to 2 weeks.

INGREDIENTS

- 2 ½ cups of regular rolled oats
- 1/3 cup of coarsely chopped almonds
- 1/8 teaspoon of kosher or sea salt
- 1/2 teaspoon of ground cinnamon
- 1/2 cup of chopped dried apricots
- 2 tablespoons of ground flaxseed
- 1/4 cup of honey
- 1/4 cup of extra-virgin olive oil
- 2 teaspoons of vanilla extract

NUTRITIONAL FACTS

- Calories: 337 Cal,
- Fat: 17 g,
- Sodium: 23 mg,
- Carbohydrates: 42 g,
- Fiber: 6 g,
- Protein: 7 g

GREEK YOGURT PARFAITS WITH ROASTED GRAPES

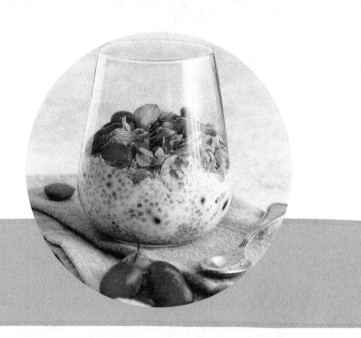

PREP. TIME: 5' - COOK TIME: 25' - SERVINGS: 4

INGREDIENTS

- 1 ½ pounds of seedless grapes (about 4 cups)
- 1 tablespoon of extra-virgin olive oil
- 2 cups of 2% plain Greek yogurt
- 1/2 cup of chopped walnuts
- 4 teaspoons of honey

NUTRITIONAL FACTS

- Calories: 300 Cal,
- Fat: 17 g,
- Cholesterol: 16 mg,
- Sodium: 59 mg,
- Carbohydrates: 34 g,
- Protein: 7g

DIRECTIONS

01 Place a large, rimmed baking sheet in the oven. Preheat the oven to 450°F with the pan inside. Wash the grapes and remove from the stems. Dry on a clean kitchen towel, and put in a bowl. Drizzle with the oil, and toss to coat.

02 Carefully remove the hot pan from the oven, and pour the grapes onto the pan. Bake for 20 to 23 minutes, until slightly wilted, stirring once halfway through.

03 Remove the baking sheet from the oven and cool on a wire rack for 5 minutes. While the grapes are cooling, assemble the parfaits by spooning the yogurt into four bowls or tall glasses. Top each bowl or glass with 2 tablespoons of walnuts and 1 teaspoon of honey.

04 When the grapes are slightly cooled, top each parfait with a quarter of the grapes. Scrape any accumulated sweet grape juice onto the parfaits and serve.

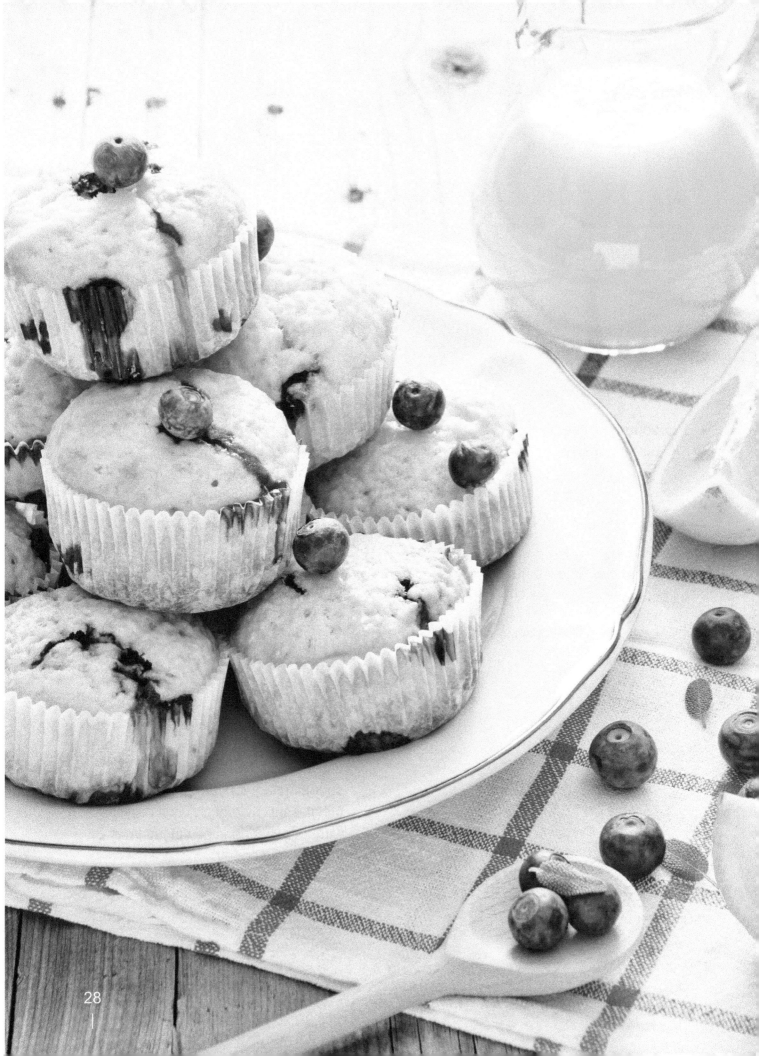

WHOLE-WHEAT BLUEBERRY MUFFINS

PREP. TIME: 5' - COOK TIME: 25' - SERVINGS: 8

DIRECTIONS

01 Preheat the oven to 375°F.
In a large bowl, mix the milk, applesauce, maple syrup, and vanilla.

02 Stir in the flour and baking soda until no dry flour is left and the batter is smooth. Gently fold in the blueberries until they are evenly distributed throughout the batter.

03 In a muffin tin, fill 8 muffin cups three-quarters full of batter.
Bake for 25 minutes, or until you can stick a knife into the center of a muffin and it comes out clean. Allow to cool before serving.

04 Tip: Both frozen and fresh blueberries will work great in this recipe. The only difference will be that muffins using fresh blueberries will cook slightly quicker than those using frozen.

INGREDIENTS

- 1/2 cup plant-based milk
- 1/2 cup unsweetened applesauce
- 1/2 cup maple syrup
- 1 teaspoon vanilla extract
- 2 cups whole-wheat flour
- 1/2 teaspoon baking soda
- 1 cup blueberries

NUTRITIONAL FACTS

- Fat: 1 g,
- Carbohydrates: 45 g,
- Fiber: 2 g,
- Protein: 4 g

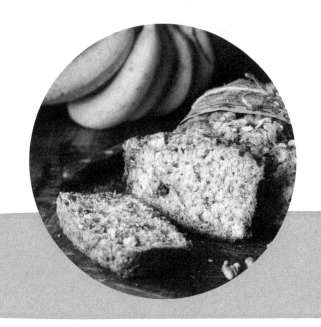

WALNUT CRUNCH BANANA BREAD

PREP. TIME: 5' - COOK TIME: 1H 30' - SERVINGS: 2

DIRECTIONS

01 Preheat the oven to 350°F.
In a large bowl, use a fork or mixing spoon to mash the bananas until they reach a puréed consistency (small bits of banana are acceptable). Stir in the maple syrup, apple cider vinegar, and vanilla.

02 Stir in the flour, cinnamon, and baking soda. Fold in the walnut pieces (if using).

03 Gently pour the batter into a loaf pan, filling it no more than three-quarters of the way full. Bake for 1 hour, or until you can stick a knife into the middle and it comes out clean.

04 Remove from the oven and allow cooling on the countertop for a minimum of 30 minutes before serving.

INGREDIENTS

- 4 ripe bananas
- 1/4 cup of maple syrup
- 1 tablespoon of apple cider vinegar
- 1 teaspoon of vanilla extract
- 1 ½ cups of whole-wheat flour
- 1/2 teaspoon of ground cinnamon
- 1/2 teaspoon of baking soda
- 1/4 cup of walnut pieces (optional)

NUTRITIONAL FACTS

- Fat: 1g,
- Carbohydrates: 40 g,
- Fiber: 5 g,
- Protein: 4 g

MUSHROOM QUICKIE SCRAMBLE

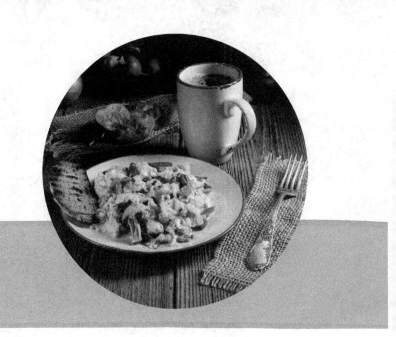

PREP. TIME 10' - COOK TIME 10' - SERVINGS 4

INGREDIENTS

- 3 small-sized eggs, whisked
- 4 pieces Bella mushrooms
- ½ cup of spinach
- ¼ cup of red bell peppers
- 1 tablespoon of ghee or coconut oil
- Salt & pepper to taste

DIRECTIONS

01 Chop the ham and veggies.
Put half a tablespoon of butter in a frying pan and heat until melted.

02 In another frying pan, heat the remaining butter.
Add the whisked eggs into the second pan while stirring continuously to avoid overcooking

03 When the eggs are done, sprinkle with salt & pepper to taste.
Mix well.
Remove from burner and transfer to a plate.
Serve and enjoy.

NUTRITIONAL FACTS

- Calories: 350
- Total Fat: 29 g
- Protein: 21 g
- Total Carbs: 5 g

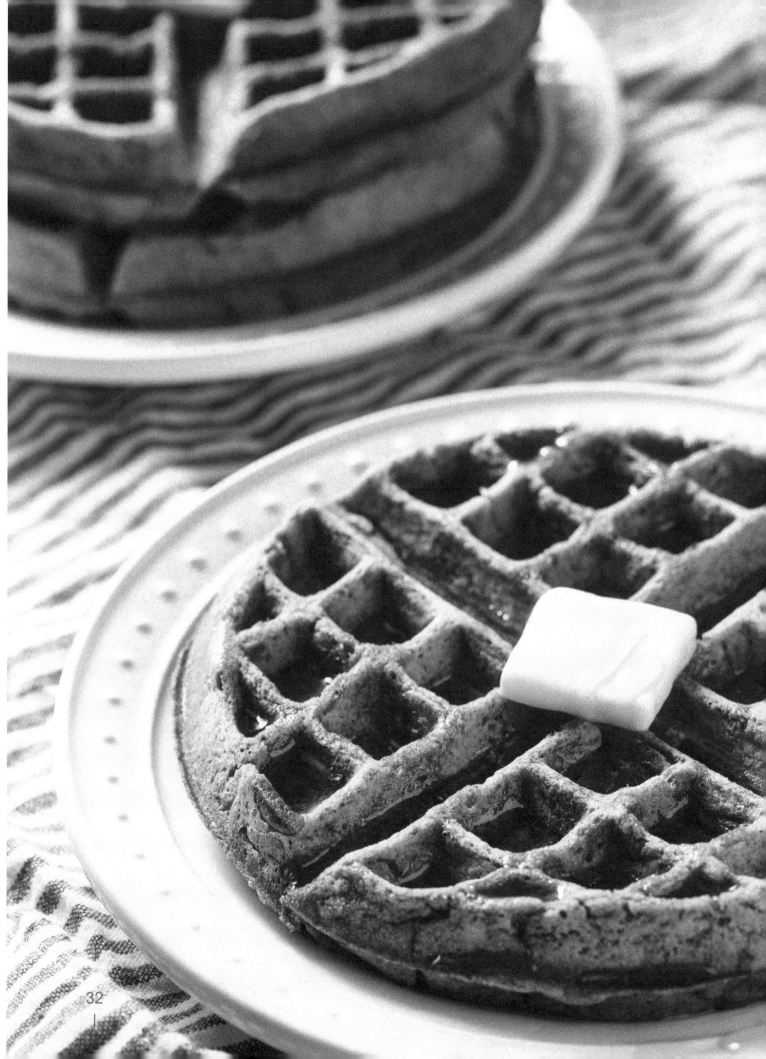

YUMMY GREEN WAFFLES

DIRECTIONS

01 Turn the waffle maker on.
In a bowl mix all the listed ingredients very well until incorporated.

02 Once the waffle maker is hot, distribute the waffle mixture into the insert.
Let cook for about 9 minutes, flipping at 6 minutes.

03 Remove from waffle maker and set aside.
Repeat the previous steps with the rest of the batter until done (should come out to 4 waffles).
Serve and enjoy!

INGREDIENTS

- 3 cups raw cauliflower, grated
- 1 cup cheddar cheese
- 1 cup mozzarella cheese
- ½ cup parmesan
- 1/3 cup chives, finely sliced
- 6 eggs
- 1 teaspoon garlic powder
- 1 teaspoon onion powder
- ½ teaspoon chili flakes
- Dash of salt and pepper

NUTRITIONAL FACTS

- Calories: 390
- Fat: 28g
- Carbs: 6g
- Fiber: 2g
- Protein: 30g

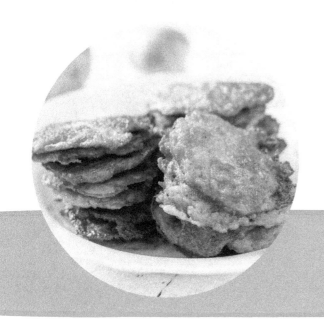

CABBAGE HASH BROWNS

PREP. TIME: 10' - COOK TIME: 10' - SERVINGS: 2

DIRECTIONS

01 Crack the egg in a bowl, add garlic powder, black pepper, and salt, whisk well, then add cabbage, toss until well mixed, and shape the mixture into four patties.

02 Take a large skillet pan, place it over medium heat, add oil, and when hot, add patties in it and cook for 3 minutes per side until golden brown.

03 Transfer hash browns to a plate and serve.

INGREDIENTS

- 1 ½ cup shredded cabbage
- 1/2 teaspoon garlic powder
- 1 egg
- 1 tablespoon coconut oil
- ½ teaspoon salt
- 1/8 teaspoon ground black pepper

NUTRITIONAL FACTS

- 336 Calories;
- 16 g Protein;
- 0.9 g Net Carb;
- 0.8 g Fiber;

COCONUT COFFEE AND GHEE

INGREDIENTS

- ½ tablespoon of coconut oil
- ½ tablespoon of ghee
- 1 to 2 cups of preferred coffee (or rooibos or black tea, if preferred)
- 1 tablespoon of coconut or almond milk

DIRECTIONS

01 Place the almond (or coconut) milk, coconut oil, ghee, and coffee in a blender (or milk frother).

02 Mix for around 10 seconds or until the coffee turns creamy and foamy.

03 Pour contents into a coffee cup. Serve immediately and enjoy!

NUTRITIONAL FACTS

- Calories: 150
- Total Fat: 15 g
- Protein: 0 g
- Total Carbs: 0 g
- Net Carbs: 0 g

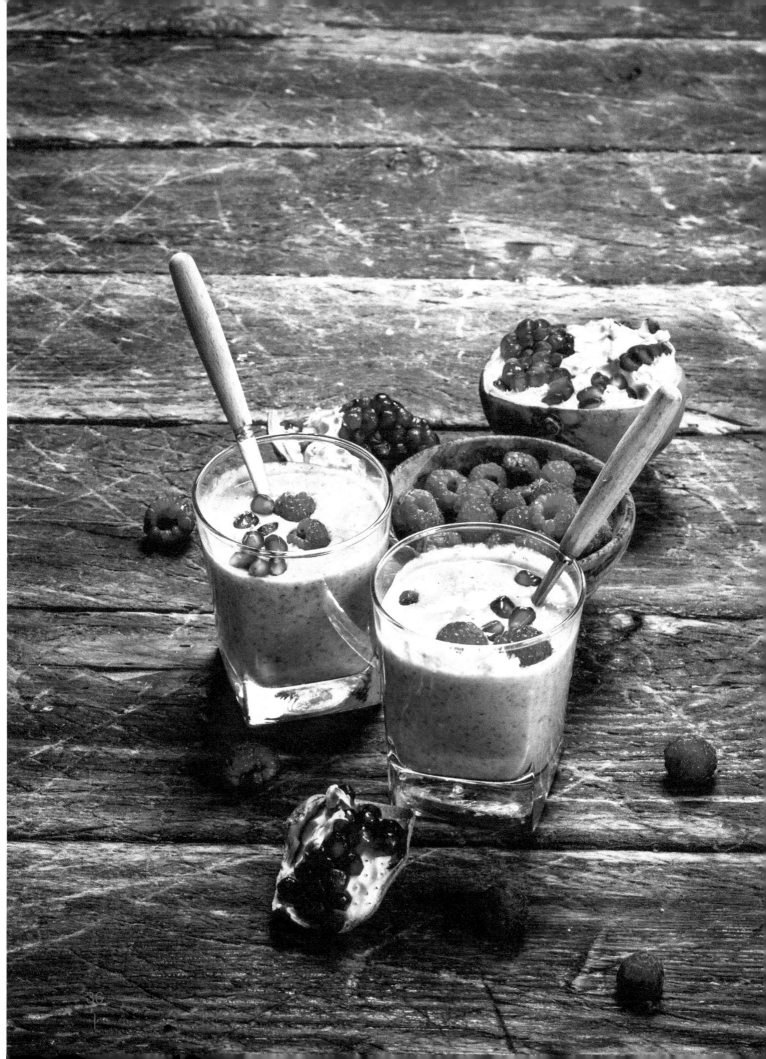

CREAMY RASPBERRY POMEGRANATE SMOOTHIE

PREP. TIME: 5' - COOK TIME: 5' - SERVINGS: 2

DIRECTIONS

01 In a blender, combine the pomegranate juice and coconut milk. Add the protein powder and spinach.

02 Add the raspberries, banana, and lemon juice, then top it off with ice. Blend until smooth and frothy.

INGREDIENTS

- 1½ cups pomegranate juice
- ½ cup unsweetened coconut milk
- 1 scoop vanilla protein powder (plant-based if you need it to be dairy-free)
- 1 cup frozen raspberries
- 1 frozen banana
- 1 to 2 tablespoons freshly compressed lemon juice
-

NUTRITIONAL FACTS

- Calories: 303
- Total fat: 3g
- Cholesterol: 0mg
- Protein: 15g
- Sodium: 165mg

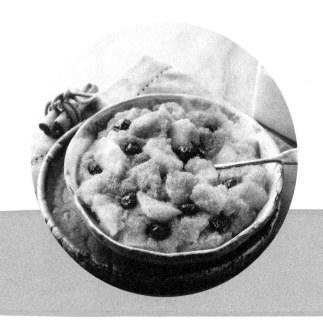

AMARANTH PORRIDGE

PREP. TIME: 5' - COOK TIME: 30' - SERVINGS: 2

DIRECTIONS

01 In a saucepan, mix in the milk with water then boil the mixture.
Stir in the amaranth then reduce the heat to medium.

02 Cook on medium heat then simmer for at least 30 minutes as you stir it occasionally.

02 Turn off the heat.
Add in cinnamon and coconut oil then stir. Serve.

INGREDIENTS

- 2 cups coconut milk
- 2 cups alkaline water
- 1 cup amaranth
- 2 tablespoons coconut oil
- 1 tablespoon ground cinnamon

NUTRITIONAL FACTS

- Calories: 434 kcal
- Fat: 35g
- Carbs: 27g
- Protein: 6.7g

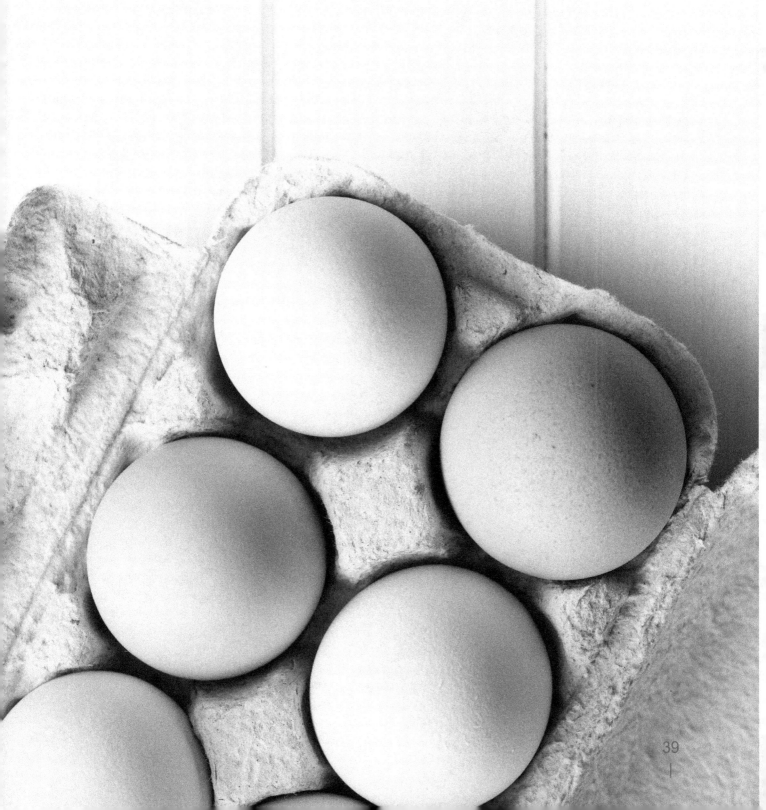

EGGS

BROCCOLI, ASPARAGUS AND CHEESE FRITTATA

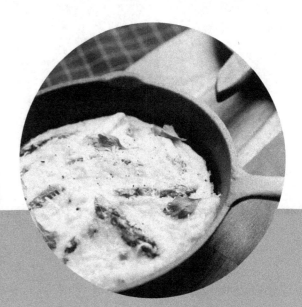

PREP. TIME: 5' - COOK TIME: 16' - SERVINGS: 2

INGREDIENTS

- ¼ cup chopped broccoli florets
- 1-ounce asparagus spear cuts
- ½ teaspoon garlic powder
- 2 tablespoon whipping cream
- 2 eggs
- 2 teaspoon tablespoon avocado oil
- 1/8 teaspoon salt
- 1/8 teaspoon ground black pepper

NUTRITIONAL FACTS

- Calories 206
- Fats 17g
- Protein 10g
- Net Carb 2 g
- Fiber 1g

DIRECTIONS

01 Turn on the oven, then set it to 350 degrees F and let it preheat.
Take a medium bowl, crack eggs in it, add salt, black pepper, and cream, whisk until combined, and then stir in cheese, set aside until required.

02 Take a medium skillet pan, place it over medium heat, add oil and when hot, add broccoli florets and asparagus, sprinkle with garlic powder, stir until mixed and cook for 3 to 4 minutes until tender.

03 Spread the vegetables evenly in the pan, pour egg mixture over them and cook for 1 to 2 minutes until the mixture begins to firm.

04 Transfer the pan into the oven and then cook for 10 to 12 minutes until frittata has cooked and the top has turned golden brown.
When done, cut the frittata into slices and then serve.

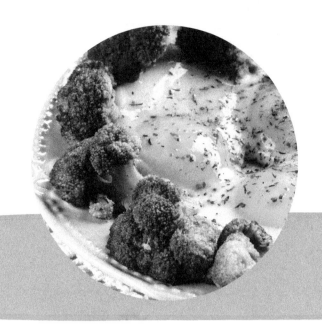

BROCCOLI AND EGG PLATE

PREP. TIME: 5' · COOK TIME: 5' · SERVINGS: 2

DIRECTIONS

01 Take a microwave-safe bowl, place broccoli florets in it, cover with a plastic wrap, microwave for 2 minutes, and then drain well.

02 Take a medium skillet pan, place it over medium heat, add oil and when hot, add broccoli florets and cook for 2 minutes until golden brown.

03 Spread broccoli florets evenly in the pan. Crack eggs in the pan, sprinkle with salt and black pepper, cover with the lid and cook for 2 to 3 minutes until eggs have cooked to the desired level.
Serve.

INGREDIENTS

- 3 oz broccoli florets, chopped
- 2 eggs
- 1 tablespoon avocado oil
- ¼ teaspoon salt
- 1/8 teaspoon ground black pepper

NUTRITIONAL FACTS

- Calories 155
- Fats 12g
- Protein 8g
- Net Carb 1.6g
- Fiber 1g

RADISH WITH FRIED EGGS

INGREDIENTS

- ½ bunch of radishes, diced
- ½ teaspoon garlic powder
- 1 tablespoon butter
- 1 tablespoon avocado oil
- 2 eggs
- 1/3 teaspoon salt
- ¼ teaspoon ground black pepper

DIRECTIONS

01 Take a medium skillet pan, place it over medium heat, add butter and when it melts, add radish, sprinkle with garlic powder and ¼ teaspoon salt and cook for 5 minutes until tender.

02 Distribute radish between two plates, then return pan over medium heat, add oil and when hot, crack eggs in it and fry for 2 to 3 minutes until cooked to the desired level.
Add eggs to the radish and then serve.

NUTRITIONAL FACTS

- 187 Calories 187
- 17 g Fats 17g
- 7 g Protein 7g
- 0.4 g Net Carb 0.4g
- 0.5 g Fiber 0.5g

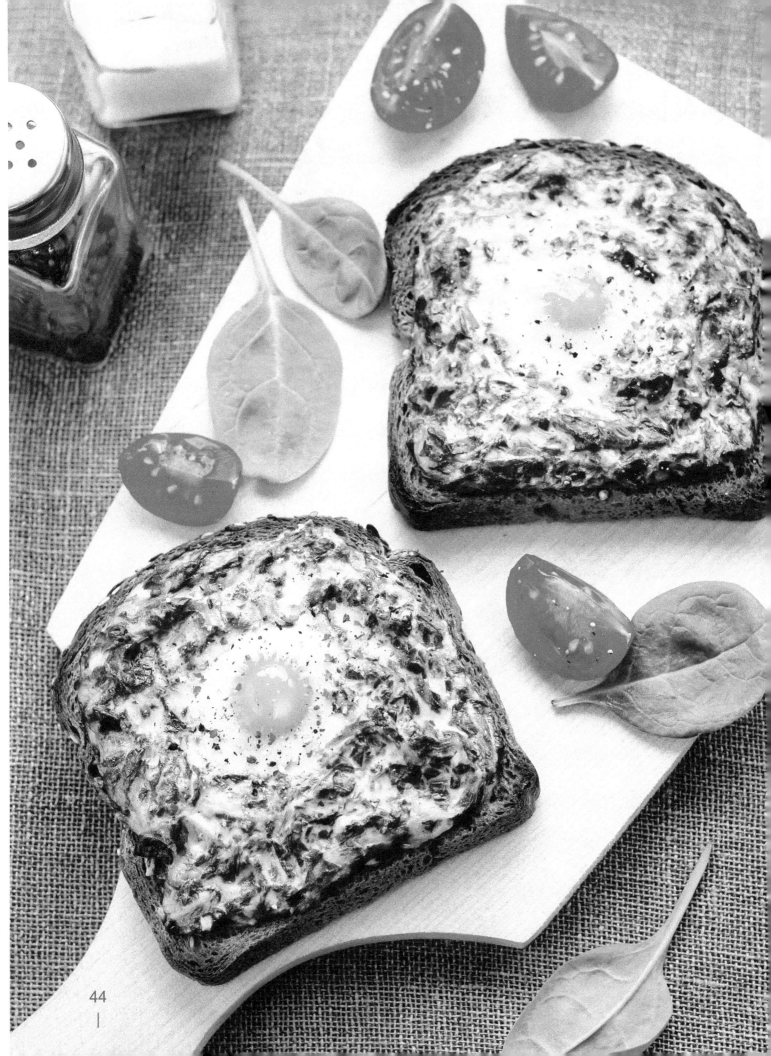

SUNNY SIDE UP EGGS ON CREAMED SPINACH

DIRECTIONS

01 Take a medium skillet pan, place it over high heat, pour in water to cover its bottom, then add spinach, toss until mixed, and cook for 2 minutes until spinach wilts.

02 Then drain the spinach by passing it through a sieve placed on a bowl and set it aside.Take a medium saucepan, place it over medium heat, add spinach, mustard, thyme, and cream, stir until mixed and cook for 2 minutes.

03 Then sprinkle black pepper over spinach, stir until mixed and remove the pan from heat.

03 Take a medium skillet pan, place it over medium-high heat, add oil and when hot, crack eggs in it and fry for 3 to 4 minutes until eggs have cooked to the desired level. Divide spinach mixture evenly between two plates, top with a fried egg and then serve.

INGREDIENTS

- 4 oz of spinach leaves
- 1 tablespoon mustard paste
- 4 tablespoon whipping cream
- 2 eggs
- ¼ teaspoon salt
- ¼ teaspoon ground black pepper
- ½ teaspoon dried thyme
- 1 tablespoon avocado oil

NUTRITIONAL FACTS

- Calories 280
- Fats 23.3g
- Protein 10.2g
- Net Carb 2.7g
- Fiber 2.8g

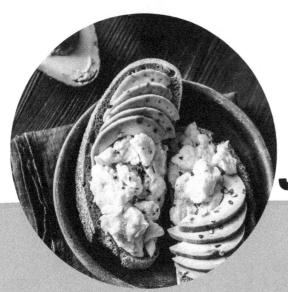

EGG SANDWICHES WITH CILANTRO-JALAPEÑO SPREAD

PREP. TIME: 20' - COOK TIME: 10' - SERVINGS: 2

DIRECTIONS

01 <u>To make the cilantro and jalapeño spread:</u>
In a food processor, combine the cilantro, jalapeño, oil, pepitas, garlic, lime juice, and salt. Whirl until smooth. Refrigerate if making in advance; otherwise set aside.

02 <u>To make the eggs:</u>
In a medium bowl, whisk the eggs, milk, and salt.
Dissolve the butter in a skillet over low heat, swirling to coat the bottom of the pan. Pour in the whisked eggs. Cook until they begin to set then, using a heatproof spatula, push them to the sides, allowing the uncooked portions to run into the bottom of the skillet. Continue until the eggs are set.

03 <u>To assemble the sandwiches:</u>
Toast the bed and spread with butter.
Spread a spoonful of the cilantro-jalapeño spread on each piece of toast. Top each with scrambled eggs.
Arrange avocado over each sandwich

INGREDIENTS

- 1 cup cilantro leaves and stems
- 1 jalapeño pepper, seeded and roughly chopped
- ½ cup extra-virgin olive oil
- ¼ cup hulled pumpkin seeds
- 2 garlic cloves, thinly sliced
- 1 tablespoon lime juice
- 1 teaspoon kosher salt
- 4 large eggs
- ¼ cup milk
- ¼ to ½ teaspoon kosher salt
- 2 tablespoons butter
- 2 slices bread
- 1 tablespoon butter
- 1 avocado

NUTRITIONAL FACTS

- Calories: 711
- Total fat: 4g
- Cholesterol: 54mg
- Fiber: 12g
- Protein: 12g
- Sodium: 327mg

CREAMY KALE BAKED EGGS

PREP. TIME: 10' - COOK TIME: 20' - SERVINGS: 2

INGREDIENTS

- 1 bunch of kale, chopped
- 1-ounce grape tomatoes halved
- 3 tablespoon whipping cream
- 2 tablespoon sour cream
- 2 eggs
- ½ teaspoon salt
- ½ teaspoon ground black pepper
- ½ teaspoon Italian seasoning
- 1 ½ tablespoon butter, unsalted

NUTRITIONAL FACTS

- Calories 301.5g
- Fats 25.5g
- Protein 9.8g
- Net Carb 4.3g
- Fiber 4g

DIRECTIONS

01 Turn on the oven, then set it to 400 degrees F and let it preheat. Meanwhile, take a medium skillet pan, place butter in it, add butter and when it melts, add kale and cook for 2 minutes until wilted

02 Add Italian seasoning, 1/3 teaspoon each of salt and black pepper, cream and sour cream, then stir until mixed and cook for 2 minutes until cheese has melted and the kale has thickened slightly.

03 Take two ramekins, divide creamed kale evenly between them, then top with cherry tomatoes and carefully crack an egg into each ramekin.

04 Sprinkle remaining salt and black pepper on eggs and then bake for 15 minutes until eggs have cooked completely.
Serve.

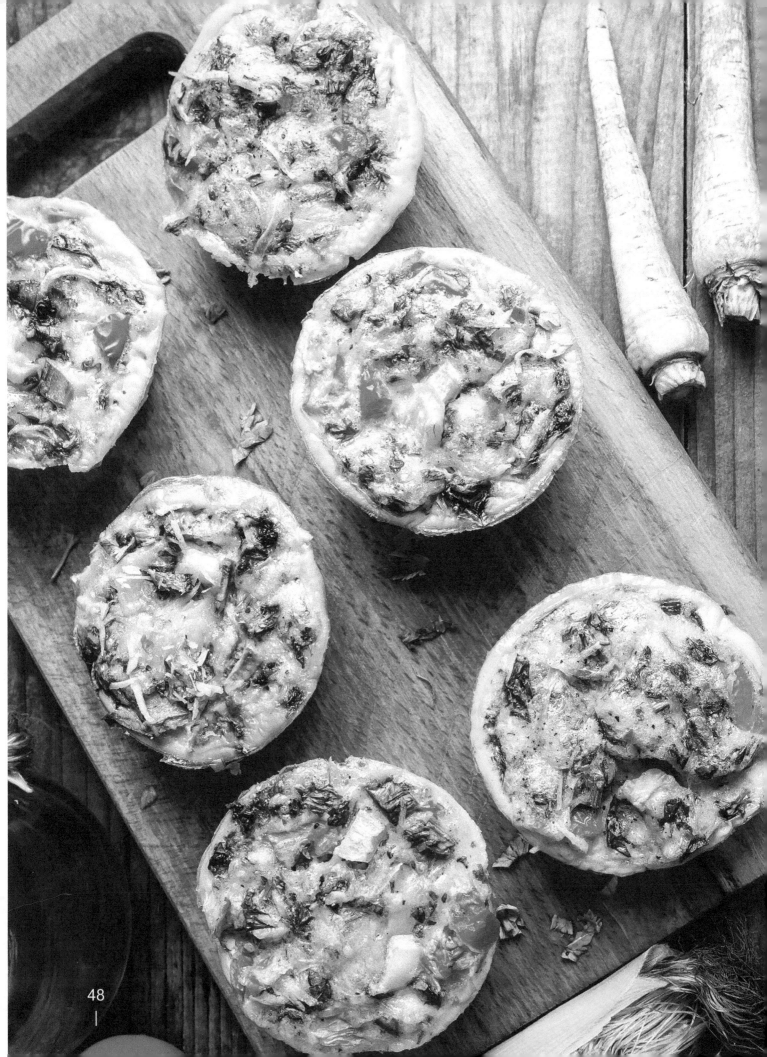

KALE, TOMATO AND GOAT CHEESE EGG MUFFINS

DIRECTIONS

01 Preheat oven to 375° F.
Whisk together the eggs, egg whites, Greek yogurt, goat cheese, and salt in a large bowl, until well mixed.

02 Stir in the kale and cherry tomatoes.
Divide mixture evenly among 20 to 24 slots of two, standard-size, lightly-greased muffin tins.
Bake for 20 to 25 minutes, until set in the middle and a knife inserted into the center comes out clean.

03 Tip: Make these on the weekend, and freeze for the week ahead. Simply pop in the microwave for 1 to 2 minutes to reheat!

INGREDIENTS

- 9 eggs
- 1 cup liquid egg whites
- 3/4 cup plain, low-fat Greek yogurt
- 2 oz crumbled goat cheese
- ½ tsp salt
- 1, 10-oz package frozen, chopped kale, thawed and patted dry
- 2 cups chopped cherry tomatoes
- Cooking spray

NUTRITIONAL FACTS

- Calories 290
- Fats 15g
- Protein 29g
- Net Carb 11g

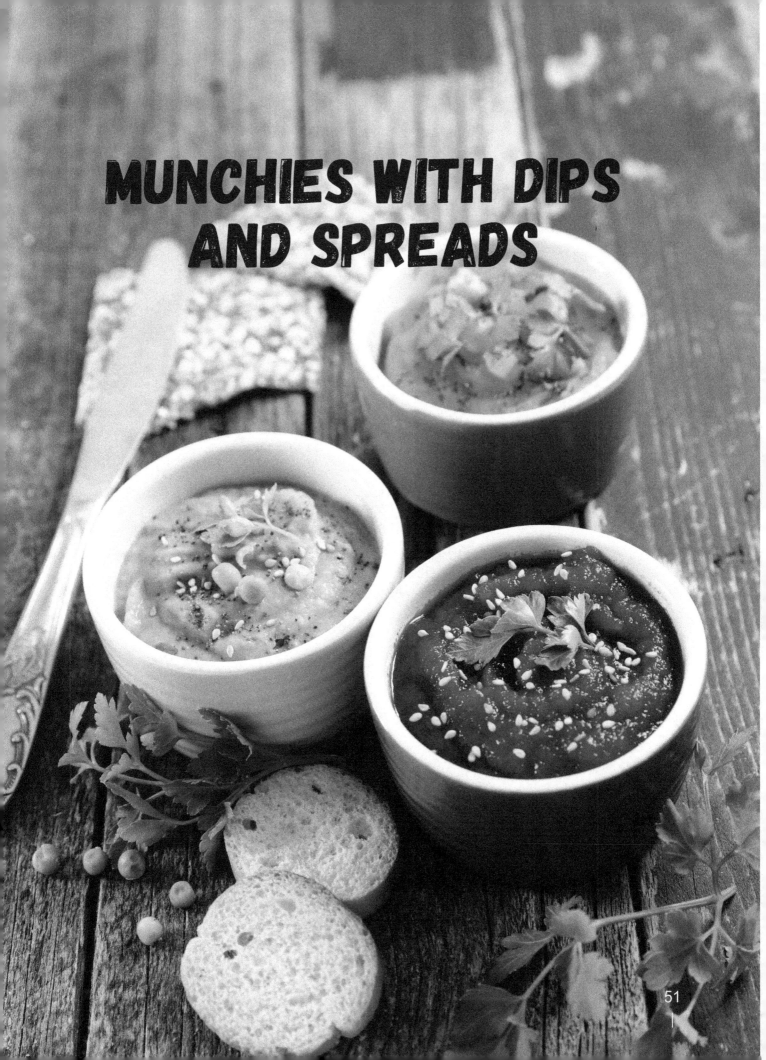

MUNCHIES WITH DIPS AND SPREADS

WHITE BEAN DIP

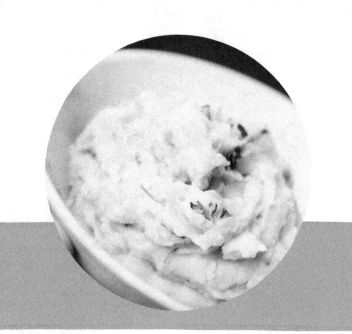

INGREDIENTS

- 15 ounces canned white beans, drained and rinsed
- 6 ounces canned artichoke hearts, drained and quartered
- 4 garlic cloves, minced
- 1 tablespoon basil, chopped
- 2 tablespoons olive oil
- Juice of ½ lemon
- Zest of ½ lemon, grated
- Salt and black pepper to the taste

DIRECTIONS

01 In your food processor, combine the beans with artichokes and rest of the ingredients, except oil, and pulse well.

02 Add the oil gradually, pulse the mix again, divide into cups, and serve as a party dip.

NUTRITIONAL FACTS

- Calories 274
- Fat 11.7 g
- Fiber 6.5 g
- Carbs 18.5 g
- Protein 16.5 g

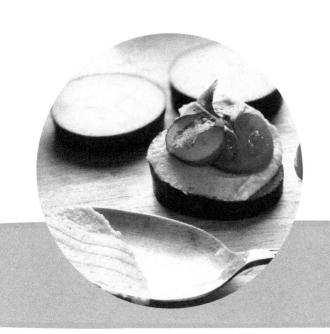

CUCUMBER BITES

PREP. TIME: 10' - COOK TIME: 0' - SERVINGS: 10

DIRECTIONS

01 Spread the hummus on each cucumber round, divide the tomato halves on each, sprinkle the cheese and parsley over it, and serve as an appetizer.

INGREDIENTS

- 1 English cucumber, sliced into 32 rounds
- 10 ounces hummus
- 16 cherry tomatoes, halved
- 1 tablespoon parsley, chopped
- 1-ounce feta cheese, crumbled

NUTRITIONAL FACTS

- Calories 162
- Fat 3.4 g
- Fiber 2 g
- Carbs 6.4 g
- Protein 2.4 g

OLIVES AND CHEESE STUFFED TOMATOES

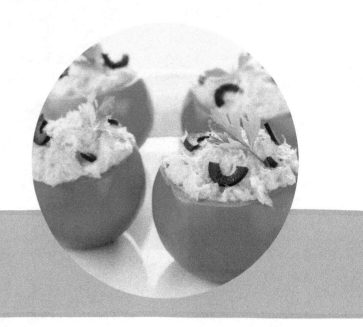

PREP. TIME: 10' - COOK TIME: 0' - SERVINGS: 8

INGREDIENTS

- 24 cherry tomatoes, top cut off, and insides scooped out
- 2 tablespoons olive oil
- ¼ teaspoon red pepper flakes
- ½ cup feta cheese, crumbled
- 2 tablespoons black olive paste
- ¼ cup mint, torn

DIRECTIONS

01 In a bowl, mix the olives paste with the rest of the ingredients except the cherry tomatoes and whisk well.

02 Stuff the cherry tomatoes with this mix, arrange them all on a platter, and serve as an appetizer.

NUTRITIONAL FACTS

- Calories 136
- Fat 8.6 g

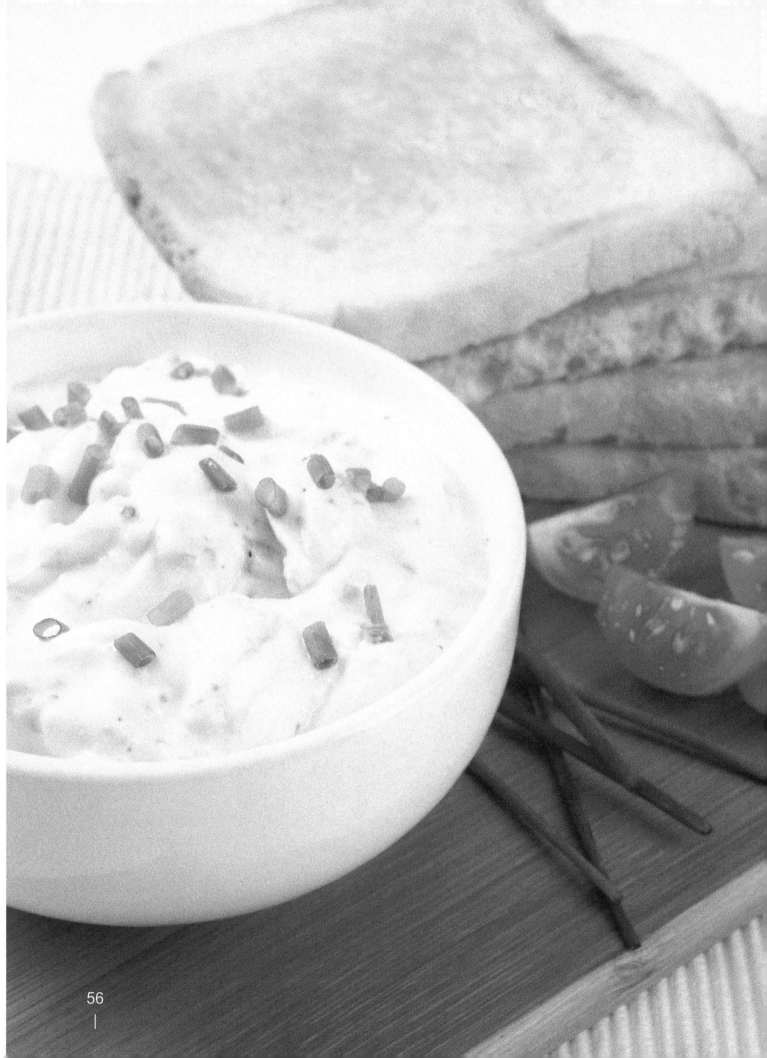

GOAT CHEESE AND CHIVES SPREAD

DIRECTIONS

01 Mix the goat cheese with the cream and the rest of the ingredients in a bowl, and whisk really well.

02 Keep in the fridge for 10 minutes and serve as a party spread.

INGREDIENTS

- 2 ounces goat cheese, crumbled
- ¾ cup sour cream
- 2 tablespoons chives, chopped
- 1 tablespoon lemon juice
- Salt and black pepper to the taste
- 2 tablespoons extra-virgin olive oil

NUTRITIONAL FACTS

- Calories 220
- Fat 11.5 g
- Fiber 4.8 g
- Carbs 8.9 g
- Protein 5.6 g

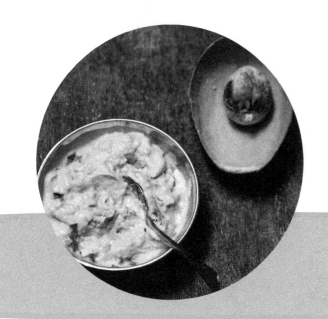

AVOCADO DIP

DIRECTIONS

01 Pour the cream with the avocados and the rest of the ingredients in a blender, and pulse well. Divide the mix into bowls and serve cold as a party dip.

INGREDIENTS

- ½ cup heavy cream
- 1 green chili pepper, chopped
- Salt and pepper to taste
- 4 avocados, pitted, peeled, and chopped
- 1 cup cilantro, chopped
- ¼ cup lime juice

NUTRITIONAL FACTS

- Calories 200
- Fat 14.5 g
- Fiber 3.8 g
- Carbs 8.1 g
- Protein 7.6 g

TOMATO SALSA

INGREDIENTS

- 1 garlic clove, minced
- 4 tablespoons olive oil
- 5 tomatoes, cubed
- 1 tablespoon balsamic vinegar
- ¼ cup basil, chopped
- 1 tablespoon parsley, chopped
- 1 tablespoon chives, chopped
- Salt and black pepper to the taste
- Pita chips for serving

DIRECTIONS

01 Mix the tomatoes with the garlic in a bowl. Add all other ingredients except pita chips; stir, divide into small cups and serve with the pita chips on the side.

NUTRITIONAL FACTS

- Calories 160
- Fat 13.7 g
- Fiber 5.5 g
- Carbs 10.1 g
- Protein 2.2

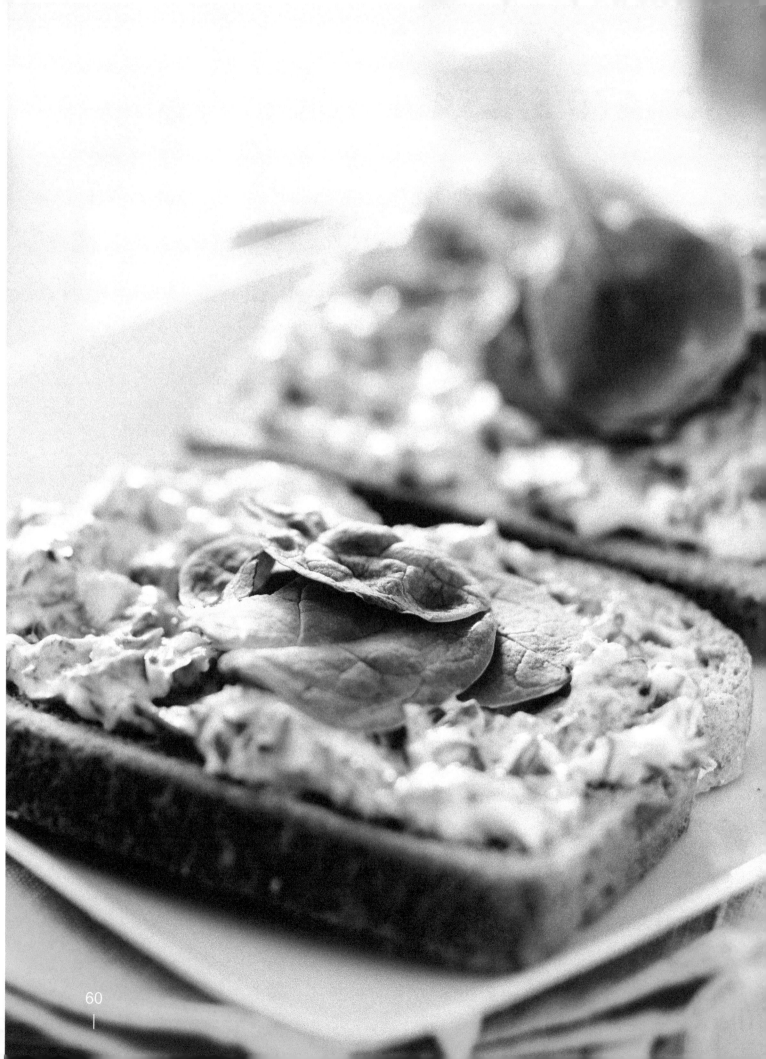

CREAMY SPINACH AND SHALLOTS DIP

DIRECTIONS

01 Combine the spinach with the shallots and the rest of the ingredients in a blender and pulse well. Divide into small bowls and serve as a party dip.

INGREDIENTS

- 1-pound spinach, roughly chopped
- 2 shallots, chopped
- 2 tablespoons mint, chopped
- ¾ cup cream cheese, soft
- Salt and black pepper to the taste

NUTRITIONAL FACTS

- Calories 204
- Fat 11.5 g
- Fiber 3.1 g
- Carbs 4.2 g
- Protein 5.9 g

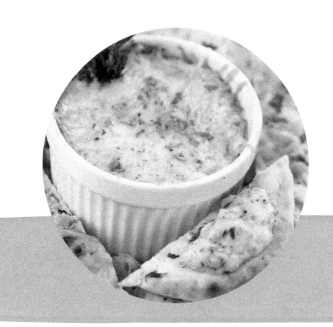

FETA ARTICHOKE DIP

PREP. TIME: 10' - COOK TIME: 30' - SERVINGS: 8

DIRECTIONS

01 In the food processor, mix the artichokes with the basil and the rest of the ingredients, pulse well, and transfer to a baking dish, then bake for 30 minutes at 350 degrees F.

INGREDIENTS

- 8 ounces artichoke hearts, drained and quartered
- ¾ cup basil, chopped
- ¾ cup green olives, pitted and chopped
- 1 cup parmesan cheese, grated
- 5 ounces feta cheese, crumbled

NUTRITIONAL FACTS

- Calories 186
- Fat 12.4 g
- Fiber 0.9 g
- Carbs 2.6 g
- Protein 1.5 g

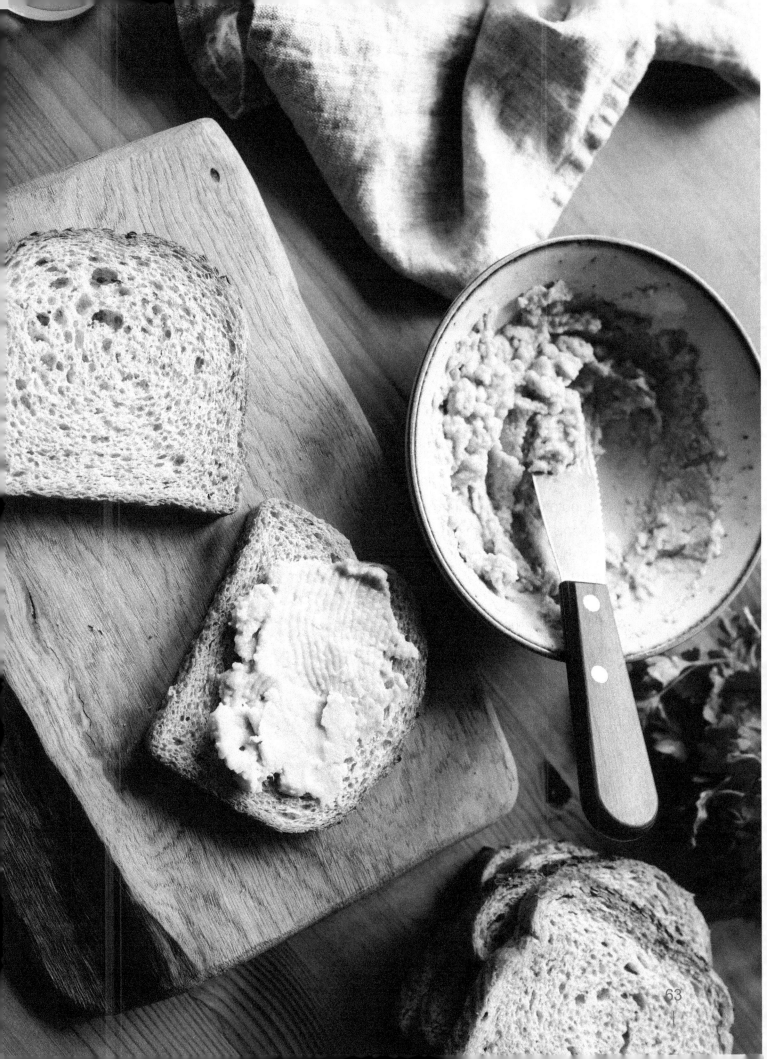

MASHED CHICKPEA, FETA, AND AVOCADO TOAST

PREP. TIME: 10' - COOK TIME: 15' - SERVINGS: 4

DIRECTIONS

01 Put the chickpeas in a large bowl. Scoop the avocado flesh into the bowl.

02 With a potato masher or large fork, mash the ingredients together until the mix has a spreadable consistency. It doesn't need to be smooth.

03 Add the feta, lemon juice, and pepper, and mix well.

04 Evenly divide the mash into the four pieces of toast and spread with a knife. Drizzle with honey and serve.

INGREDIENTS

- 1 (15-ounce) can of chickpeas, drained and rinsed
- 1 avocado, pitted
- 1/2 cup of diced feta cheese (about 2 ounces)
- 2 teaspoons of freshly squeezed lemon juice or 1 tablespoon orange juice
- 1/2 teaspoon of freshly ground black pepper
- 4 pieces of multigrain toast
- 2 teaspoons of honey

NUTRITIONAL FACTS

- Calories: 337 Cal
- Fat: 13 g
- Sodium: 564 mg
- Carbohydrates: 43 g
- Fiber: 12 g
- Protein: 13 g

SALADS

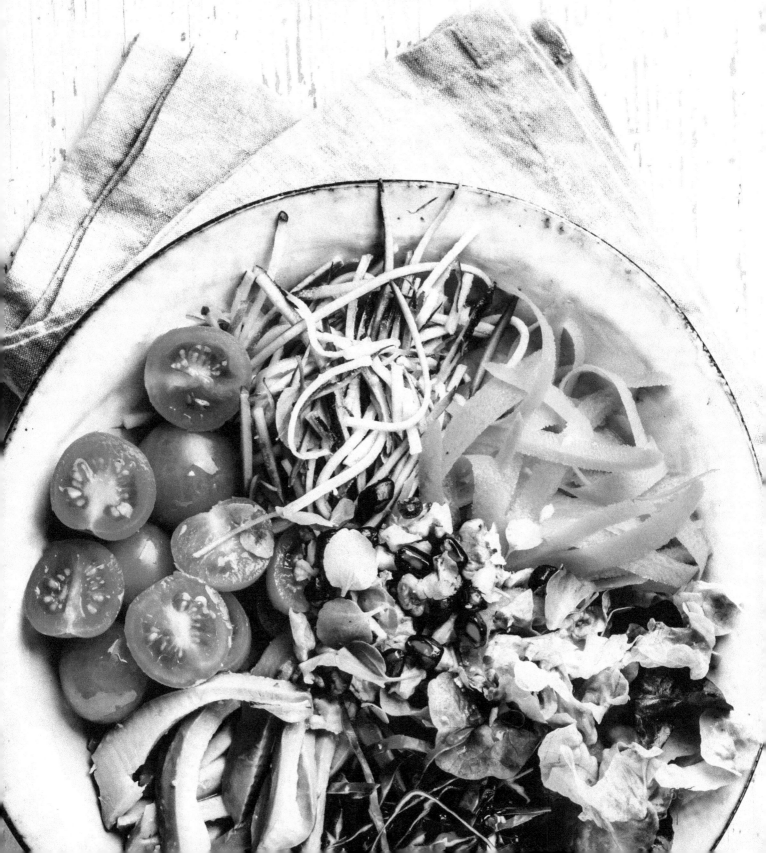

FENNEL AND ARUGULA SALAD

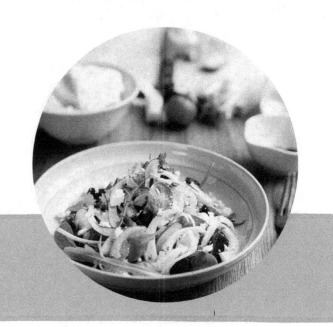

PREP. TIME: 10' - COOK TIME: 0' - SERVINGS: 2

INGREDIENTS

- 5 ounces washed and dried arugula
- 1 small fennel bulb, it can be either shaved or tiny sliced.
- 2 tablespoons extra virgin oil or any cooking oil
- 1 teaspoon lemon zest
- 1/2 teaspoon salt
- Pepper (freshly ground)
- Pecorino

DIRECTIONS

01 Mix the arugula and shaved fennel in a serving bowl.

02 In another bowl, mix the olive oil or cooking oil, lemon zest, salt and pepper. Shake together until it becomes creamy and smooth.

03 Pour and dress over the salad, tossing gently for it to combine.
Peel or shave out some slices of pecorino and put it on top of the salad
Serve immediately

NUTRITIONAL FACTS

- Protein: 2.1 g,
- Carbohydrates: 14.3 g,
- Dietary Fiber: 3.4 g,
- Sugars: 9.1 g,
- Fat: 9.7 g

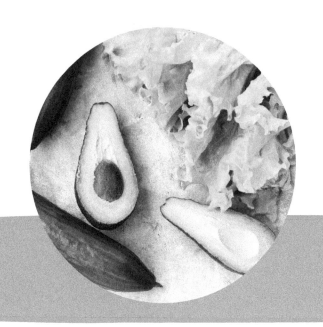

SALAD SANDWICHES

PREP. TIME: 5' - COOK TIME: 0' - SERVINGS: 2

DIRECTIONS

01 Rinse the lettuce leaves, pat dry with a paper towel, and then smear each leaf with butter.

02 Top lettuce with cheese and avocado and serve.

INGREDIENTS

- 1 medium avocado, peeled, pitted, diced
- 2 leaves of iceberg lettuce
- 1-ounce unsalted butter
- 2-ounce cheddar cheese, sliced

NUTRITIONAL FACTS

- 187 Calories;
- 17 g Fats;
- 5 g Protein;
- 4 g Net Carb;
- 1.5 g Fiber;

VEGAN RECIPES

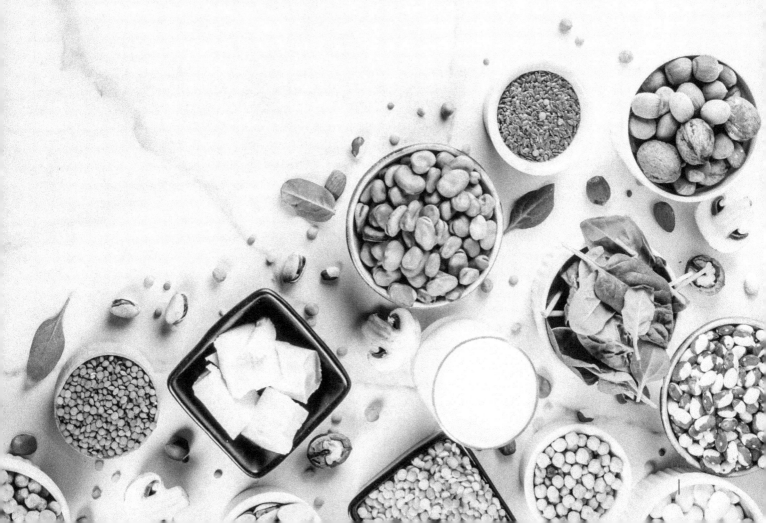

COCONUT PANCAKES

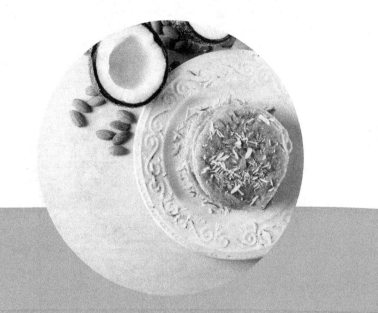

PREP. TIME: 5' - COOK TIME: 15' - SERVINGS: 4

INGREDIENTS

- 1 cup coconut flour
- 2 tablespoons arrowroot powder
- 1 teaspoon baking powder
- 1 cup coconut milk
- 3 tablespoons coconut oil

DIRECTIONS

01 In a medium container, mix in all the dry ingredients.
Add the coconut milk and 2 tablespoons of the coconut oil then mix properly.

02 In a skillet, melt 1 teaspoon of coconut oil.
Pour a ladle of the batter into the skillet then swirl the pan to spread the batter evenly into a smooth pancake.

03 Cook it for around 3 minutes on medium heat, until it becomes firm.
Turn the pancake to the other side then cook it for another 2 minutes until it turns golden brown.
Cook the remaining pancakes in the same manner.
Serve.

NUTRITIONAL FACTS

- Calories: 377 kcal
- Fat: 14.9g
- Carbs: 60.7g
- Protein: 6.4g

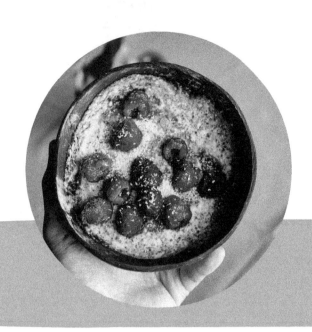

CRUNCHY QUINOA MEAL

PREP. TIME: 5' · COOK TIME: 25' · SERVINGS: 2

DIRECTIONS

01 In a saucepan, pour milk and bring it to a boil over moderate heat.
Add the quinoa to the milk and then bring it to a boil once more.

02 Let it simmer for at least 15 minutes on medium heat until the milk is reduced. Stir in the cinnamon then mix properly.

03 Cover and cook for 8 minutes until the milk is completely absorbed.

04 Add the raspberry and cook the meal for 30 seconds.
Serve and enjoy.

INGREDIENTS

- 3 cups coconut milk
- 1 cup rinsed quinoa
- 1/8 teaspoon ground cinnamon
- 1 cup raspberry
- 1/2 cup chopped coconuts

NUTRITIONAL FACTS

- Calories: 271 kcal
- Fat: 3.7g
- Carbs: 54g
- Proteins: 6.5g

JACKFRUIT VEGETABLE FRY

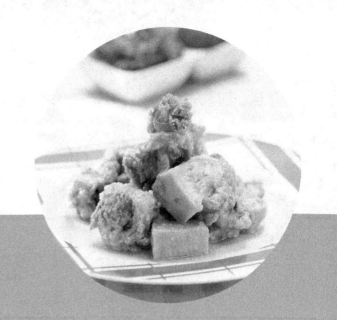

PREP. TIME: 5' - COOK TIME: 5' - SERVINGS: 6

INGREDIENTS

- 2 finely chopped small onions
- 2 cups finely chopped cherry tomatoes
- 1/8 teaspoon ground turmeric
- 1 tablespoon olive oil
- 2 seeded and chopped red bell peppers
- 3 cups seeded and chopped firm jackfruit
- 1/8 teaspoon cayenne pepper
- 2 tablespoons chopped fresh basil leaves
- Salt

DIRECTIONS

01 In a greased skillet, sauté the onions and bell peppers for about 5 minutes.
Add the tomatoes and stir.

02 Cook for 2 minutes.
Then add the jackfruit, cayenne pepper, salt, and turmericup.

03 Cook for about 8 minutes.
Garnish the meal with basil leaves.
Serve warm.

NUTRITIONAL FACTS

- Calories: 236 kcal
- Fat: 1.8g
- Carbs: 48.3g
- Protein: 7g

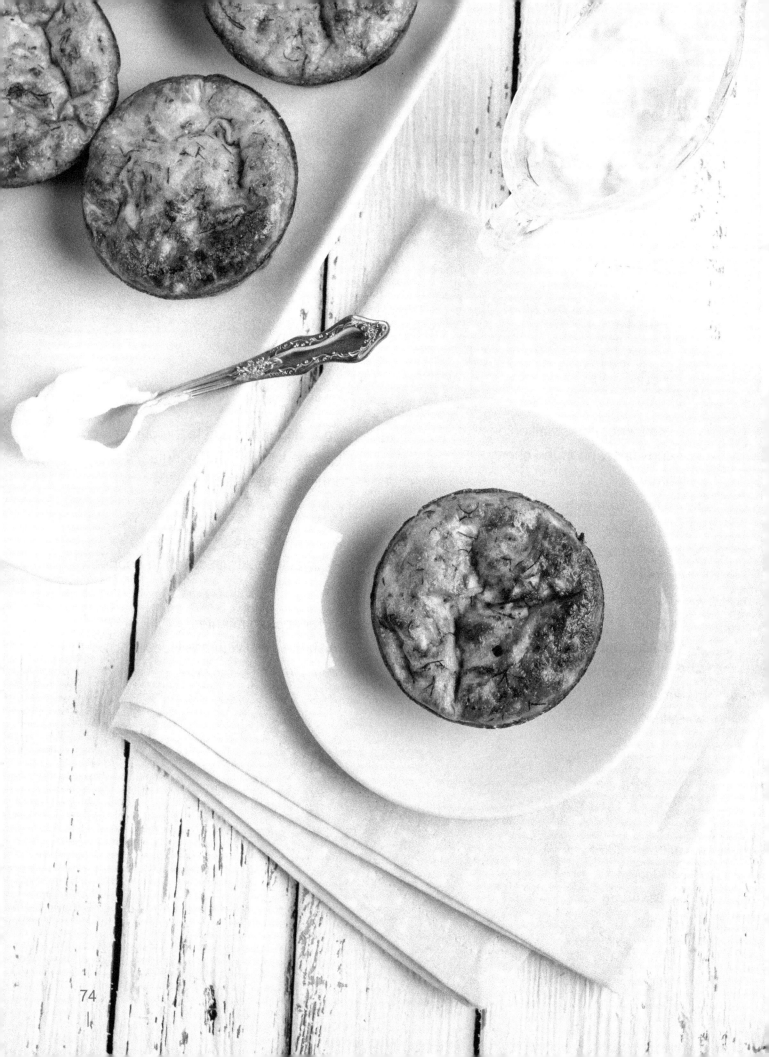

ZUCCHINI MUFFINS

DIRECTIONS

01 Tune the temperature of your oven to 375ºF. Grease the muffin tray with the cooking spray.

02 In a bowl, mix the flaxseed with water. In a glass bowl, mash the bananas then stir in the remaining ingredients.

03 Properly mix and then divide the mixture into the muffin tray. Bake it for 25 minutes. Serve.

INGREDIENTS

- 1 tablespoon ground flaxseed
- 3 tablespoons alkaline water
- 1/4 cup walnut butter
- 3 medium over-ripe bananas
- 2 small grated zucchinis
- 1/2 cup coconut milk
- 1 teaspoon vanilla extract
- 2 cups coconut flour
- 1 tablespoon baking powder
- 1 teaspoon cinnamon
- 1/4 teaspoon sea salt

NUTRITIONAL FACTS

- Calories: 127 kcal
- Fat: 6.6g
- Carbs: 13g
- Protein: 0.7g

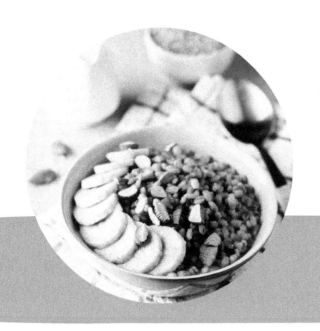

BANANA BARLEY PORRIDGE

PREP. TIME: 15' · COOK TIME: 5' · SERVINGS: 2

DIRECTIONS

01 In a bowl, properly mix barley with half of the coconut milk and stevia. Cover the mixing bowl then refrigerate for about 6 hours.

02 In a saucepan, mix the barley mixture with coconut milk. Cook for about 5 minutes on moderate heat.

03 Then top it with the chopped coconuts and the banana slices. Serve.

INGREDIENTS

- 1 cup divided unsweetened coconut milk
- 1 small peeled and sliced banana
- 1/2 cup barley
- 3 drops liquid stevia
- 1/4 cup chopped coconuts

NUTRITIONAL FACTS

- Calories: 159kcal
- Fat: 8.4g
- Carbs: 19.8g
- Proteins: 4.6g

PUMPKIN SPICE QUINOA

PREP. TIME: 10' - COOK TIME: 0' - SERVINGS: 2

INGREDIENTS

- 1 cup cooked quinoa
- 1 cup unsweetened coconut milk
- 1 large mashed banana
- 1/4 cup pumpkin puree
- 1 teaspoon pumpkin spice
- 2 teaspoons chia seeds

DIRECTIONS

01 In a container, mix all the ingredients. Seal the lid then shake the container properly to mix.

02 Refrigerate overnight. Serve.

NUTRITIONAL FACTS

- Calories: 212 kcal
- Fat: 11.9g
- Carbs: 31.7g
- Protein: 7.3g

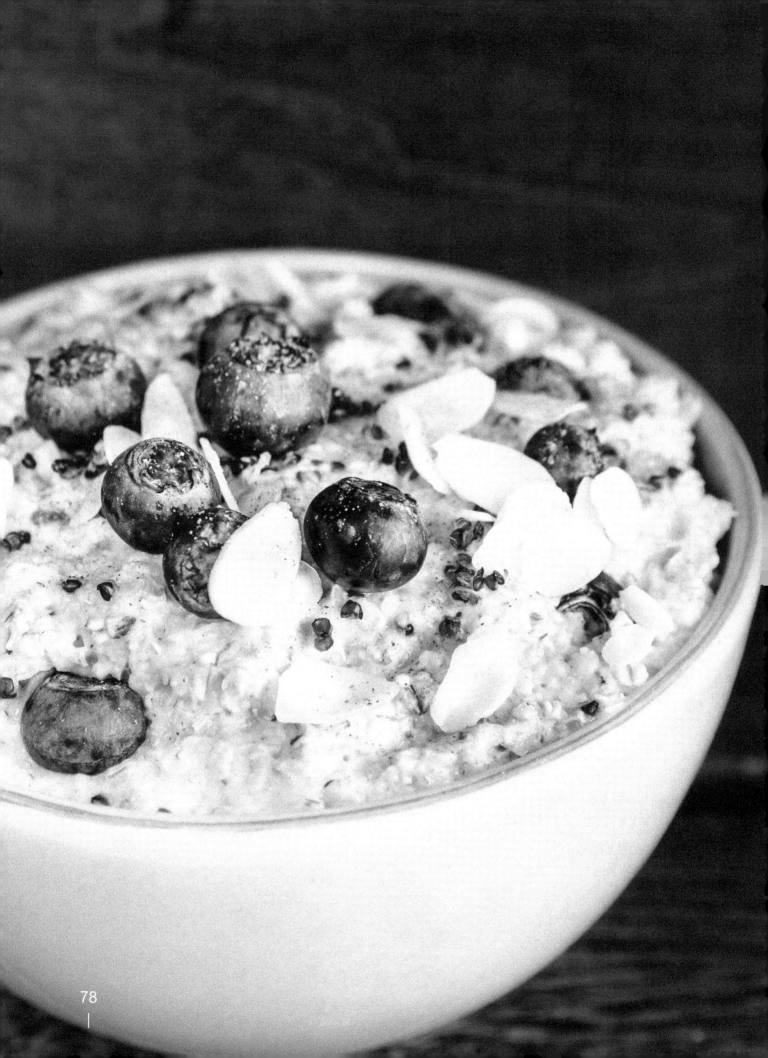

QUINOA PORRIDGE

PREP. TIME: 5' - COOK TIME: 25' - SERVINGS: 2

DIRECTIONS

01 In a saucepan, boil the coconut milk over high heat.
Add the quinoa to the milk then bring the mixture to a boil.

02 You then let it simmer for 15 minutes on medium heat until the milk is reduced.
Add the cinnamon and mix it properly in the saucepan.

03 Cover the saucepan and cook for at least 8 minutes until the milk is completely absorbed.

04 Add in the blueberries then cook for 30 more seconds.
Serve.

INGREDIENTS

- 2 cups coconut milk
- 1 cup rinsed quinoa
- 1/8 teaspoon ground cinnamon
- 1 cup fresh blueberries

NUTRITIONAL FACTS

- Calories: 271 kcal
- Fat: 3.7g
- Carbs: 54g
- Protein:6.5g

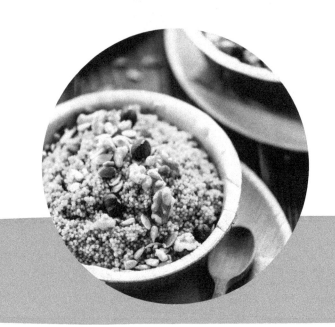

MILLET PORRIDGE

PREP. TIME: 10' · COOK TIME: 20' · SERVINGS: 2

DIRECTIONS

01 Sauté the millet in a non-stick skillet for about 3 minutes.
Add salt and water then stir.

02 Let the meal boil then reduce the amount of heat.
Cook for 15 minutes then add the remaining ingredients. Stir.

03 Cook the meal for 4 extra minutes.
Serve the meal with a topping of the chopped nuts.

INGREDIENTS

- 1 tablespoon finely chopped coconuts
- 1/2 cup unsweetened coconut milk
- 1/2 cup rinsed and drained millet
- 1-1/2 cups alkaline water
- 3 drops liquid stevia
- Sea salt

NUTRITIONAL FACTS

- Calories: 219 kcal
- Fat: 4.5g
- Carbs: 38.2g
- Protein: 6.4g

HEMP SEED PORRIDGE

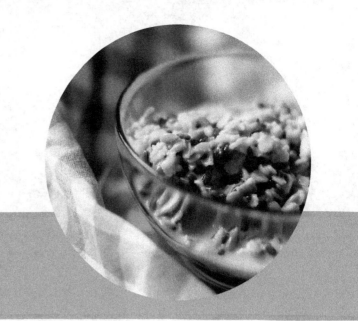

INGREDIENTS

- 3 cups cooked hemp seed
- 1 packet Stevia
- 1 cup coconut milk

DIRECTIONS

01 In a saucepan, mix the rice and the coconut milk over moderate heat for about 5 minutes as you stir it constantly.

02 Remove the pan from the burner then add the Stevia. Stir.

03 Serve in 6 bowls.
Enjoy.

NUTRITIONAL FACTS

- Calories: 236 kcal
- Fat: 1.8g
- Carbs: 48.3g
- Protein: 7g

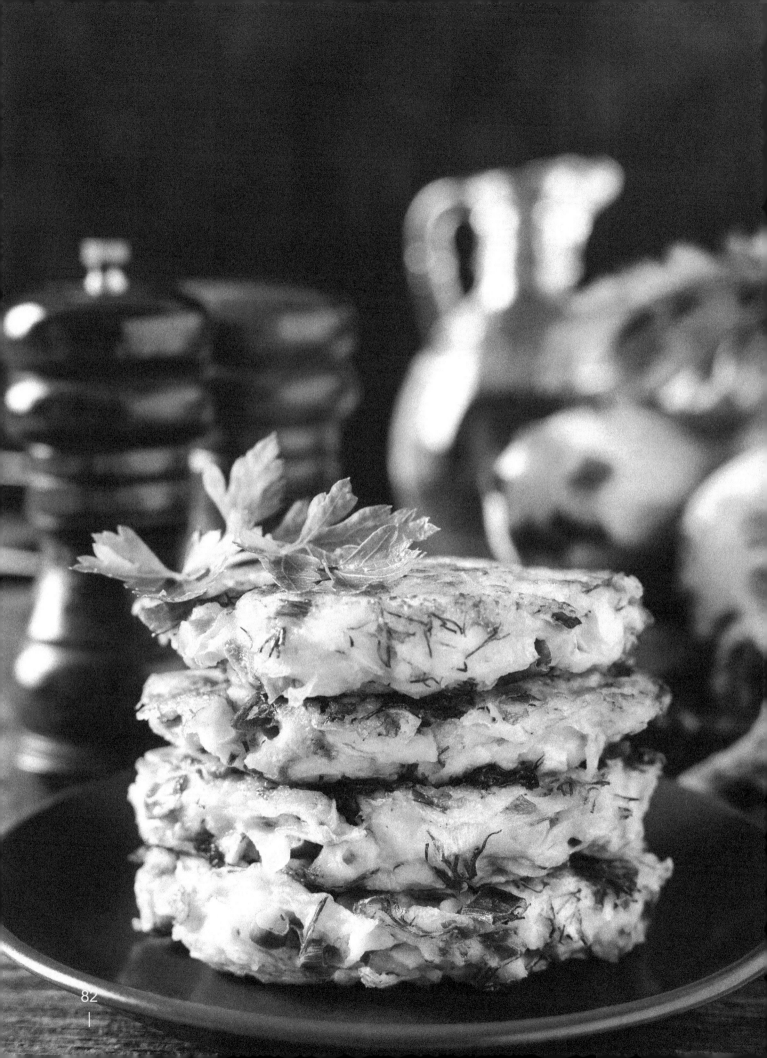

VEGGIE FRITTERS

DIRECTIONS

01 In a bowl, combine the garlic with the onions, scallions, and the rest of the ingredients except the oil, stir well and shape medium fritters out of this mix.

02 Heat oil in a pan over medium-high heat, add the fritters, cook for 5 minutes on each side, arrange on a platter and serve.

INGREDIENTS

- 2 garlic cloves, minced
- 2 yellow onions, chopped
- 4 scallions, chopped
- 2 carrots, grated
- 2 teaspoons cumin, ground
- ½ teaspoon turmeric powder
- Salt and black pepper to the taste
- ¼ teaspoon coriander, ground
- 2 tablespoons parsley, chopped
- ¼ teaspoon lemon juice
- ½ cup almond flour
- 2 beets, peeled and grated
- 2 eggs, whisked
- ¼ cup tapioca flour
- 3 tablespoons olive oil

NUTRITIONAL FACTS

- Calories 209
- Fat 11.2 g
- Fiber 3 g
- Carbs 4.4 g
- Protein 4.8 g

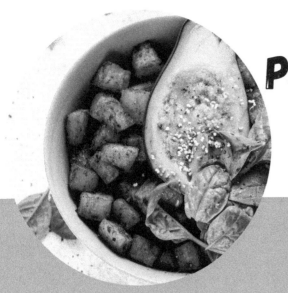

POTATO HASH WITH CILANTRO-LIME CREAM

PREP. TIME: 20' - COOK TIME: 30' - SERVINGS: 2

INGREDIENTS

For the cilantro-lime cream
- 1 avocado, halved and pitted
- ¼ cup packed fresh cilantro leaves and stems
- 2 tablespoons freshly squeezed lime juice
- 1 garlic clove, peeled
- 1 teaspoon kosher salt
- ½ teaspoon ground cumin
- 2 tablespoons extra-virgin olive oil

For the hash
- ½ teaspoon kosher salt
- 1 large sweet potato, cut into ¾-inch pieces
- 2 tablespoons extra-virgin olive oil
- 1 onion, thinly sliced
- 2 garlic cloves, crushed
- 1 red bell pepper, thinly sliced
- 1 teaspoon ground cumin
- ¼ teaspoon ground turmeric

- A pinch of freshly ground black pepper
- 2 tablespoons fresh cilantro leaves, chopped
- ½ jalapeño pepper, seeded and chopped (optional)
- Hot sauce, for serving (optional)

NUTRITIONAL FACTS

- Calories: 520
- Total fat: 43g
- Cholesterol: 0mg
- Fiber: 2g
- Protein: 12g
- Sodium: 1719mg

POTATO HASH WITH CILANTRO-LIME CREAM

DIRECTIONS

01 **To make the cilantro-lime cream:**

Add the avocado flesh in a food compressor. Add the cilantro, lime juice, garlic, salt, and cumin. Whirl until smooth. Taste and adjust seasonings, as needed. If you do not have a food processor or blender, simply mash the avocado well with a fork; the results will have more texture, but will still work. Cover and refrigerate until ready to serve.

02 **To make the hash**

Boil salt water in a medium pot over high heat. Add the sweet potato and cook for about 20 minutes until tender. Drain thoroughly.

03 Heat olive oil in a big skillet over low heat until it shimmers. Add the onion and sauté for about 4 minutes until translucent. Put the garlic and cook, turning, for about 30 seconds. Add the cooked sweet potato and red bell pepper. Season the hash with cumin, salt, turmeric, and pepper. Sauté for 5 to 7 minutes, until the sweet potatoes are golden and the red bell pepper is soft.

04 Divide the sweet potatoes between 2 bowls and spoon the sauce over them. Scatter the cilantro and jalapeño (optional) over each and serve with hot sauce (optional).

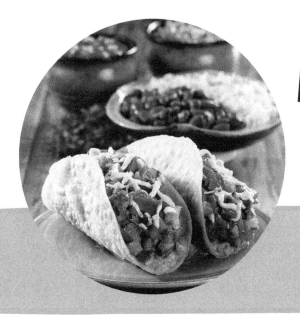

BLACK BEANS AND SWEET POTATO TACOS

PREP. TIME: 10' - COOK TIME: 30' - SERVINGS: 6

INGREDIENTS

- 1-pound sweet potato (about 2 medium teaspoons), remove skin
- 2 tablespoons of olive oil, divided
- 1 tablespoon kosar salt, divided
- ¼ teaspoon fresh black pepper on large white or yellow onion
- 2 teaspoons of red pepper
- 1 teaspoon of cumin
- 1 (15 oz.) can black beans, drained
- 1 cup of water
- ¼ cup freshly chopped garlic
- 12 pieces Corn
- Guacamole
- Sliced cheese or feta cheese
- Wood Wedge

NUTRITIONAL FACTS

- Calories: 251
- Total fat: 4g
- Cholesterol: 94mg
- Fiber: 2g
- Protein: 15g

BLACK BEANS AND SWEET POTATO TACOS

DIRECTIONS

01 In the oven, set out a tray in the middle rack and preheat to 425 degrees Fahrenheit. Set a big sheet of aluminum foil on the work surface. Collect the tortillas from the top and wrap them completely in foil. Put it aside.

02 Put sweet potatoes on a small baking sheet. Mix with one tablespoon oil and sprinkle with 1/2 teaspoon salt and 1/4 teaspoon black pepper. Mix it properly and arrange it in a single layer on the sheet. Fry for 20 minutes. Cover the potatoes with a flat lid and set aside.

03 Put the foil wrapping in the oven and continue to cook for about 10 minutes until the sweet potatoes are browned and stained and the seasonings are heated. Also, cook the beans.

04 Thereafter, heat one tablespoon oil in a large skillet over low heat. Add the onions and cook, occasionally stirring, until translucent, about 3 minutes. Mix the pepper powder, cumin, and 1/2 teaspoon salt. Add the beans and water.

05 Shield the pan and reduce the heat to low heat. Cook for 5 minutes, then slice and use the back of the fork to chop the beans a little, about half of the total. Continue cooking till the water content of the mixture is evaporated, and a semi-solid state is reached.

06 Peel the sweet potatoes and add the cantaloupe to the black beans and mix. Fill the taco cavity with a mixture of black beans and top with guacamole and cheese. Serve with lime wedges.

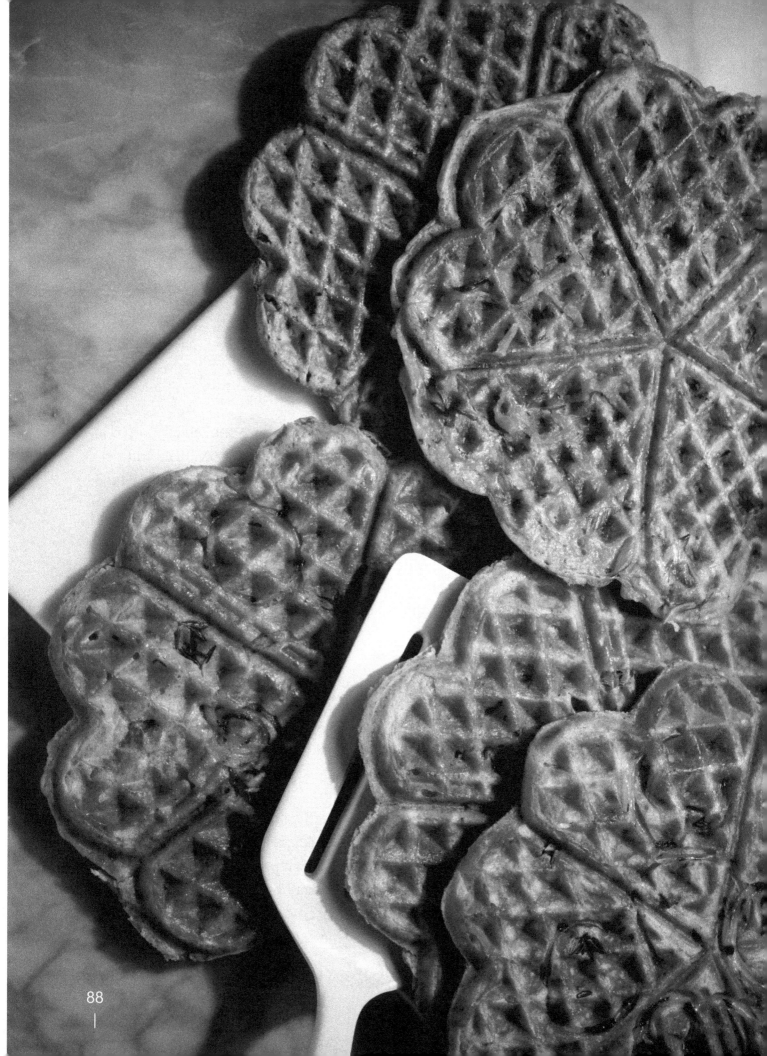

SPICY WAFFLE WITH JALAPENO

DIRECTIONS

01 Switch on a mini waffle maker and let it preheat for 5 minutes. Meanwhile, take a medium bowl, place all the ingredients in it and then mix by using an immersion blender until smooth.

02 Ladle the batter evenly into the waffle maker, shut with lid, and let it cook for 3 to 4 minutes until firm and golden brown.

INGREDIENTS

- 2 teaspoon coconut flour
- ½ tablespoon chopped jalapeno pepper
- 2 teaspoon cream cheese
- 1 egg
- 2 oz shredded mozzarella cheese
- ¼ teaspoon salt
- 1/8 teaspoon ground black pepper

NUTRITIONAL FACTS

- Calories 153
- Fats 10.7g
- Protein 11.1g
- Net Carb 1g
- Fiber 1g

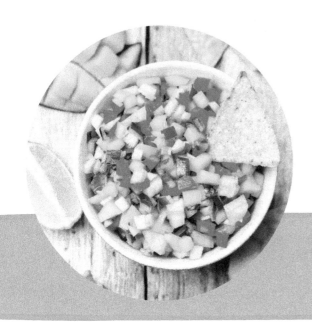

CHILI MANGO AND WATERMELON SALSA

DIRECTIONS

01 In a bowl, mix tomato with watermelon, onion, and rest of the ingredients except the pita chips and toss well.

02 Divide the mix into small cups and serve with pita chips on the side.

INGREDIENTS

- 1 red tomato, chopped
- Salt and black pepper to the taste
- 1 cup watermelon, seedless, peeled and cubed
- 1 red onion, chopped
- 2 mangos, peeled and chopped
- 2 chili peppers, chopped
- ¼ cup cilantro, chopped
- 3 tablespoons lime juice
- Pita chips for serving

NUTRITIONAL FACTS

- Calories 62
- Fat g
- Fiber 1.3 g
- Carbs 3.9 g
- Protein 2.3 g

CUCUMBER SANDWICH BITES

PREP. TIME: 5' - COOK TIME: 0' - SERVINGS: 8

INGREDIENTS

- 1 cucumber, sliced
- 8 slices whole-wheat bread
- 2 tablespoons cream cheese, soft
- 1 tablespoon chives, chopped
- ¼ cup avocado, peeled, pitted, and mashed
- 1 teaspoon mustard
- Salt and black pepper to the taste

DIRECTIONS

01 Spread the mashed avocado on each bread slice, also spread the rest of the ingredients except the cucumber slices.

02 Divide the cucumber slices on the bread slices, cut each slice in thirds, arrange on a platter and serve as an appetizer.

NUTRITIONAL FACTS

- Calories 187
- Fat 12.4 g
- Fiber 2.1 g
- Carbs 4.5 g
- Protein 8.2 g

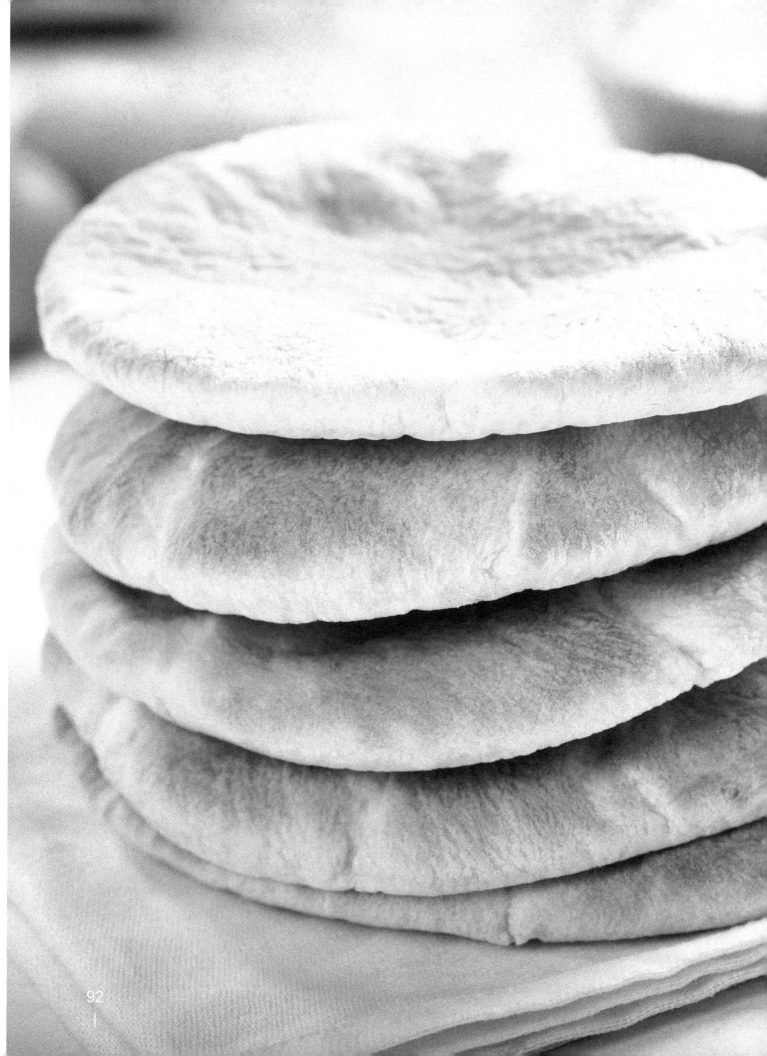

WHEAT PITA BREAD WEDGES

DIRECTIONS

01 Mix the water, yeast and honey in your mixing bowl allowing it to sit for 4 or 5 minutes.
Then add the flours, olive oil and salt, nixing it for a couple of minutes until it sticks together.
Take a little flour and sprinkle it on the surface, making a dough.

02 Add more flour if necessary, to the dough until it becomes smooth and more elastic. This might take up to 5 minutes.
Make a ball with it and cover it an oiled bowl for about an hour until it is doubled

03 Remove the dough and divide it equally into 9 parts with each part circle shaped like a ball.
Cover with a clean damp cloth.
Preheat the oven to 230C and bake for 4 to 5 minutes
Allow the homemade whole wheat pita bread to cool before serving.

INGREDIENTS

- 230 ml. (or a cup) lukewarm water
- 2 teaspoons honey
- 2 teaspoons yeast (dry)
- 1 teaspoon salt
- 1½ cup whole wheat flour (180grams)
- 1 teaspoon extra virgin oil or any cooking oil.

NUTRITIONAL FACTS

- Protein: 3.2 g
- Carbohydrates: 17.7 g
- Dietary Fiber: 2.4 g
- Sugars 0.3 g
- Fat: 5.3g

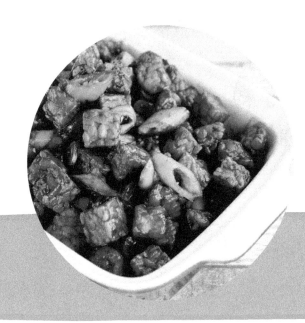

GREEN RISOTTO

PREP. TIME: 10' - COOK TIME: 30' - SERVINGS: 4

DIRECTIONS

01
Heat your oven to 400 ° C.
Cut your tempeh block into squares in bite form.
Heat coconut oil over medium to high heat in a non-stick skillet.

02
When melted and heated, add the tempeh and cook on one side for 2-4 minutes, or until the tempeh turns down into a golden-brown color.
Flip the tempeh bits, and cook for 2-4 minutes.

03
Mix the lemon juice, tamari, maple syrup, basil, water, garlic, and black pepper while tempeh is browning.
Drop the mixture over tempeh, then swirl to cover the tempeh.

03
Sauté for 2-3 minutes, then turn the tempeh and sauté 1-2 minutes more.
The tempeh, on both sides, should be soft and orange.

INGREDIENTS

- 1 packet of tempeh
- 2 to 3 teaspoons of coconut oil
- 3 tablespoons of lemon juice
- 2 teaspoons of maple syrup
- 1 to 2 teaspoons of Bragg's Liquid aminos or low-sodium tamari (optional);
- 2 teaspoons of water;
- 1/4 teaspoon of dried basil
- 1/4 teaspoon of powdered garlic;
- Black pepper (freshly grounded); to taste

NUTRITIONAL FACTS

- Carbohydrates: 22 Cal
- Fats: 17 g
- Sugar: 5 g
- Protein: 21 g
- Fiber: 9 g

HERBED WILD RICE

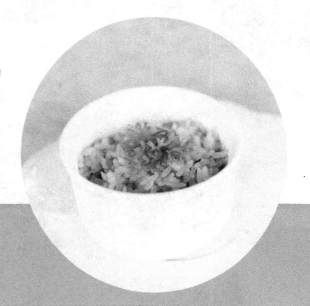

INGREDIENTS

- 3 cups wild rice, rinsed and drained
- 6 cups Roasted Vegetable Broth
- 1 onion, chopped
- 1/2 teaspoon salt
- 1/2 teaspoon dried thyme leaves
- 1/2 teaspoon dried basil leaves
- 1 bay leaf
- 1/3 cup chopped fresh flat-leaf parsley

DIRECTIONS

01 In a 6-quart slow cooker, mix the wild rice, vegetable broth, onion, salt, thyme, basil, and bay leaf.

02 Cover and cook on low for 4 to 6 hours, or until the wild rice is tender but still firm. You can cook this dish longer until the wild rice pops, taking about 5 to 6 hours.

03 Remove and discard the bay leaf. Stir in the parsley and serve.

NUTRITIONAL FACTS

- Calories: 258 Cal,
- Carbohydrates: 54 g,
- Sugar: 3 g,
- Fiber: 5 g,
- Fat: 2 g,
- Sodium: 257 mg

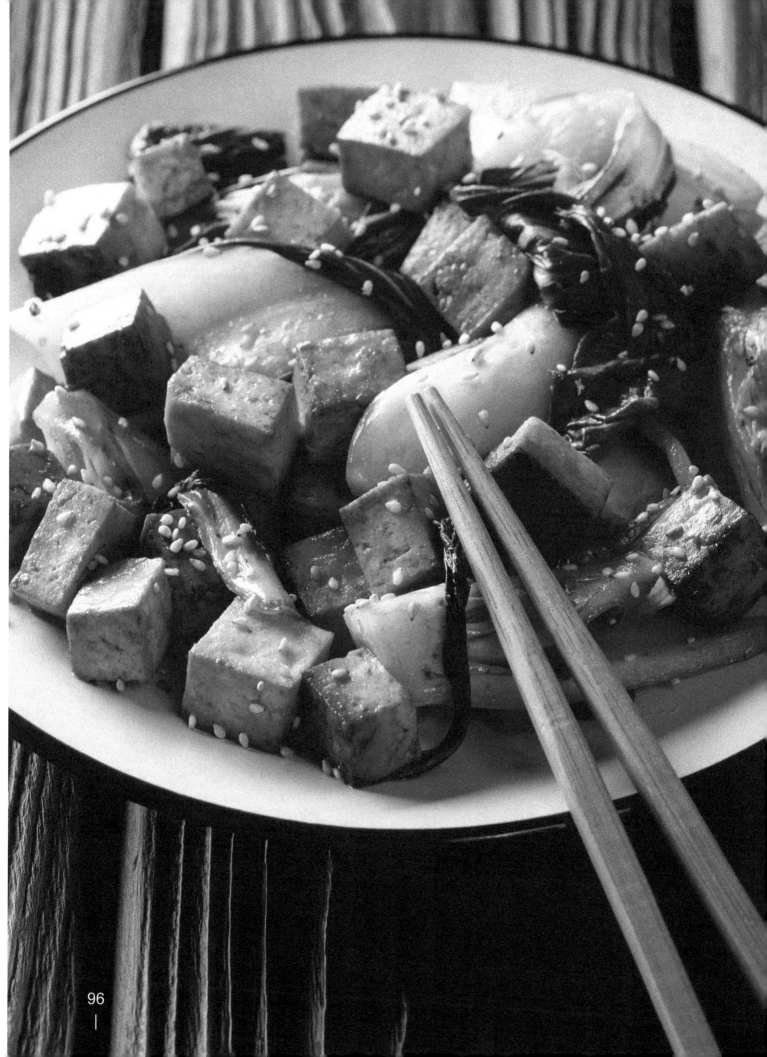

BOK CHOY WITH TOFU STIR FRY

DIRECTIONS

01 With paper towels, pat the tofu dry and cut into tiny pieces of bite-size around 1/2 inch wide.
Heat coconut oil in a wide skillet till it becomes warm.

02 Remove tofu and stir-fry until painted softly. Stir-fry for 1-2 minutes, until the choy of the Bok starts to wilt. When this occurs, apply the vegetable broth and all the remaining ingredients to the skillet.

03 Keep stir-frying until all components are well coated, and the bulk of the liquid evaporates, around 5-6 minutes.
Serve over brown rice or quinoa.

INGREDIENTS

- 1 lb. Super-firm tofu, drained and pressed
- 1 tablespoon coconut oil
- 1 clove garlic, minced
- 3 heads Baby bok choy; chopped
- Low-sodium vegetable broth
- 2 teaspoons Maple syrup
- Braggs liquid aminos
- 1 to 2 teaspoons Sambal oelek, similar chili sauce
- Scallion or green onion, chopped
- 1 teaspoon freshly grated ginger
- Quinoa/rice, for serving

NUTRITIONAL FACTS

- Calories: 263.7 Cal
- Fat 4.2 g
- Sodium: 683.6 mg
- Potassium: 313.7 mg
- Carbohydrate: 35.7 g

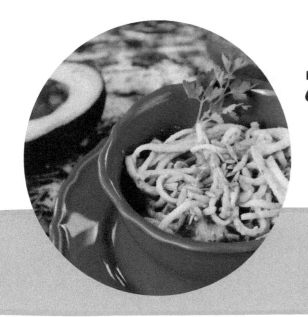

ZUCCHINI NOODLES WITH CREAMY AVOCADO PESTO

PREP. TIME: 5' - COOK TIME: 20' - SERVINGS: 4

DIRECTIONS

01 Spiralize the courgettes and set them aside on paper towels to absorb the excess water.

02 In a food processor, put avocados, lemon juice, basil leaves, garlic, pine nuts, and sea salt and pulse until chopped.
Then put olive oil in a slow stream till emulsified and creamy.

03 Drizzle olive oil in a skillet over medium-high heat and put zucchini noodles, cooking for about 2 minutes till tender.

03 Put zucchini noodles in a big bowl and toss with avocado pesto. Season with cracked pepper and a little Parmesan and serve.

INGREDIENTS

- 6 cups spiralized zucchini
- 1 tablespoon olive oil
- 6 oz. avocado
- 1 basil leaf
- 3 garlic cloves
- 1/3 oz. pine nuts
- 2 tablespoon lemon juice
- 1/2 teaspoon salt
- 1/4 teaspoon black pepper

NUTRITIONAL FACTS

- Calories: 362 Cal
- Carbohydrates: 16 g
- Protein: 4.6 g
- Fat: 34.1 g
- Sodium: 28 mg
- Sugar: 4.1 g

CELERIAC STUFFED AVOCADO

PREP. TIME: 10' - COOK TIME: 0' - SERVINGS: 2

INGREDIENTS

- 1 avocado
- 1 celery root, finely chopped
- 2 tablespoon mayonnaise
- ½ of a lemon, juiced, zested
- 2 tablespoon mayonnaise
- ¼ teaspoon salt

DIRECTIONS

01 Prepare avocado, cut it in half and then remove its pit.

02 Place remaining ingredients in a bowl, stir well until combined, and evenly stuff this mixture into avocado halves.
Serve

NUTRITIONAL FACTS

- Calories 285
- Fats 27g
- Protein 2.8g
- Net Carb 4.4g
- Fiber 2.6g

CPSIA information can be obtained
at www.ICGtesting.com
Printed in the USA
BVHW011748150521
607359BV00007B/1759

9 781802 223576